Drugs and Sports

OPPOSING VIEWPOINTS® DIGESTS

Drugs and Sports

GAIL B. STEWART

Greenhaven Press, Inc., San Diego, California

Library of Congress Cataloging-in-Publication Data

Stewart, Gail, 1949–
    Drugs and sports / Gail B. Stewart.
       p.   cm. — (Opposing viewpoints digests)
    Includes bibliographical references and index.
    Summary: Addresses opposing views on drugs and sports, including whether drug use is a serious problem in sports, whether its use should be banned, why athletes take drugs, and if they should be tested for them.
    ISBN 1-56510-749-7 (lib. bdg. : alk. paper). — ISBN 1-56510-748-9 (pbk. : alk. paper)
    1. Doping in sports—Juvenile literature. [1. Doping in sports. 2. Athletes—Drug use.] I. Title. II. Series.
RC1230.S75   1998
362.29'088'796—dc21   98-14610
                                                               CIP
                                                               AC

Cover Photo: © Jim Olive/Uniphoto
AP/Wide World: 24, 37, 66
Archive Photos: 44
North Wind Picture Archive: 9
Reuters/Archive Photos: 48 (Denis Paquin);
56 (Mike Blake); 76, 77 (Eriko Sugita)
UPI/Corbis-Bettmann: 51, 70

CONTENTS

FOREWORD

The only way in which a human being can make some approach to knowing the whole of a subject is by hearing what can be said about it by persons of every variety of opinion and studying all modes in which it can be looked at by every character of mind. No wise man ever acquired his wisdom in any mode but this.

—John Stuart Mill

Today, young adults are inundated with a wide variety of points of view on an equally wide spectrum of subjects. Often overshadowing traditional books and newspapers as forums for these views are a host of broadcast, print, and electronic media, including television news and entertainment programs, talk shows, and commercials; radio talk shows and call-in lines; movies, home videos, and compact discs; magazines and supermarket tabloids; and the increasingly popular and influential Internet.

For teenagers, this multiplicity of sources, ideas, and opinions can be both positive and negative. On the one hand, a wealth of useful, interesting, and enlightening information is readily available virtually at their fingertips, underscoring the need for teens to recognize and consider a wide range of views besides their own. As Mark Twain put it, "It were not best that we should all think alike; it is difference of opinion that makes horse races." On the other hand, the range of opinions on a given subject is often too wide to absorb and analyze easily. Trying to keep up with, sort out, and form personal opinions from such a barrage can be daunting for anyone, let alone young people who have not yet acquired effective critical judgment skills.

Moreover, to the task of evaluating this assortment of impersonal information, many teenagers bring firsthand experience of serious and emotionally charged social and health problems, including divorce, family violence, alcoholism and drug abuse, rape, unwanted pregnancy, the spread of AIDS, and eating disorders. Teens are often forced to deal with these problems before they are capable of objective opinion based on reason and judgment. All too often, teens' response to these deep personal issues is impulsive rather than carefully considered.

Greenhaven Press's Opposing Viewpoints Digests are designed to aid in examining important current issues in a way that develops critical thinking and evaluating skills. Each book presents thought-provoking argument and stimulating debate on a single issue. By examining an issue from many different points of view, readers come to realize its complexity and acknowledge the validity of opposing opinions. This insight is especially helpful in writing reports, research papers, and persuasive essays, when students must competently address common objections and controversies related to their topic. In addition, examination of the diverse mix of opinions in each volume challenges readers to question their own strongly held opinions and assumptions. While the point of such examination is not to change readers' minds, examining views that oppose their own will certainly deepen their own knowledge of the issue and help them realize exactly why they hold the opinion they do.

The Opposing Viewpoints Digests offer a number of unique features that sharpen young readers' critical thinking and reading skills. To assure an appropriate and consistent reading level for young adults, all essays in each volume are written by a single author. Each essay heavily quotes readable primary sources that are fully cited to allow for further research and documentation. Thus, primary sources are introduced in a context to enhance comprehension.

In addition, each volume includes extensive research tools. A section containing relevant source material includes interviews, excerpts from original research, and the opinions of prominent spokespersons. A "facts about" section allows students to peruse relevant facts and statistics; these statistics are also fully cited, allowing students to question and analyze the credibility of the source. Two bibliographies, one for young adults and one listing the author's sources, are also included; both are annotated to guide student research. Finally, a comprehensive index allows students to scan and locate content efficiently.

Greenhaven's Opposing Viewpoints Digests, like Greenhaven's higher level and critically acclaimed Opposing Viewpoints Series, have been developed around the concept that an awareness and appreciation for the complexity of seemingly simple issues is particularly important in a democratic society. In a democracy, the common good is often, and very appropriately, decided by open debate of widely varying views. As one of our democracy's greatest advocates, Thomas Jefferson, observed, "Difference of opinion leads to inquiry, and inquiry to truth." It is to this principle that Opposing Viewpoints Digests are dedicated.

A Brief Overview of Drug Use in Sports

Every two years since 1982, Bob Goldman, a Chicago physician specializing in sports medicine, has conducted the same survey. About two hundred subjects—all amateur athletes—are asked to respond to the following scenario: You are offered a banned performance-enhancing drug that comes with two guarantees. The first is that you will not be caught. The second is that you will win every competition you enter for the next five years, and then you will die from the side effects of the substance. Would you take the drug?

More than half of the athletes, says Goldman, respond with a "yes."

Magic Mushrooms, Sheep Testicles, and the First "Dope"

It is not much of a secret these days that some athletes will do anything, try anything, if it will give them an edge over their opponents. Although many people condemn contemporary society today for the pressure and high stakes of modern sports, in reality, athletes have been using performance-enhancing substances for many centuries.

In ancient Egypt, for example, athletes believed that if they ground the rear hooves of an Abyssinian ass, boiled them in oil, and flavored them with rose petals, the mixture would give them superhuman strength. Some early athletes ate special mushrooms that they thought would help them win. The ancient Greeks, too, had their favorite concoctions for extra strength and speed. As one former Olympic track coach jokes, "Had the

IAAF's [International Amateur Athletic Federation's] banned list been in place in ancient Greece, many an Olympic champion might have lost his laurels for ingesting sheep testicles—a prime source of testosterone."[1]

Even some of the terms we use for drug use in sports today have their roots in South Africa centuries ago. Both athletes and warriors among the Kaffi people would drink a beverage called *dop*, made from alcohol and cola, to help them feel more fierce for competition, and also to mask fatigue and pain. Over the years, an *e* was added to *dop*, and its meaning was expanded to include any substance taken by an athlete with the intention of improving performance.

The Beginnings of Doping Today

Modern drug use in sports became more prevalent during the middle of the nineteenth century. The first documented doping

Ancient athletes sometimes used performance-enhancing drugs during competitions. Ground hooves of an Abyssinian ass boiled in oil and flavored with rose petals were believed to give the athlete who drank the concoction superhuman strength.

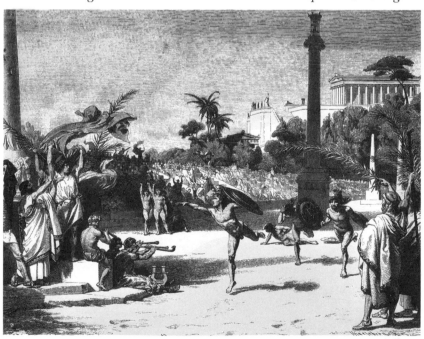

incident took place in Amsterdam in 1865, when it was discovered that Dutch swimmers were taking stimulants to mask the pain of exhausted muscles, allowing them to put out greater effort for longer amounts of time.

Many of the drugs athletes were using were potentially dangerous. Runners experimented with a drug called nitroglycerin, reasoning that since the drug causes the coronary arteries to dilate, the wider arteries might let more blood reach the heart. Although they hoped the result would be a faster pace, most ended up with splitting headaches.

Cyclists, too, invented concoctions for extra energy. The most dangerous of these was the "speedball," a combination of heroin and cocaine that was supposed to increase endurance. A cross-country cyclist died from taking a speedball in 1886; this was the first drug-related death documented in athletics.

The instances of doping became more common as time went on. European cyclists used large amounts of caffeine and ether-coated sugar cubes to mask pain and fatigue. Russian speed skaters used poisons such as arsenic and strychnine as stimulants; boxers drank brandy laced with cocaine. Historians note that this particular drink was also used by U.S. Olympic marathoner Thomas Hicks, who won a gold medal in 1904.

The Birth of Steroids

But stimulants such as these make up only one segment of the drugs used to enhance athletic performance. More than forty years ago, the athletic world found another type of drug that seems to work miracles by creating muscle mass in an astonishingly short amount of time, enabling athletes to improve speed, power, and strength. These drugs are known as steroids, called "'roids" by many users.

Simply put, steroids pack on muscle, which is an athlete's biggest asset. One Olympic expert explains the way the drugs work in the body:

It heightens RNA activity, and spurs the synthesis of protein, the basic component of muscle, bone, and skin. It helps muscles to regenerate more quickly from the stress of training, in order to be stressed again. And for sprinters and other athletes in power events, the drug excites the motor neurons in their muscle fibres, resulting in faster muscle contractions—the foundation for higher speed and improved reaction times.[2]

The first steroids were developed by German scientists during World War II. Steroids—derived from the male hormone testosterone—were given to Nazi troops to increase their muscle strength and make them more aggressive in battle. Ironically, steroids were extensively used after the war to rebuild the wasted bodies of those who had survived Nazi concentration camps.

After the war, weight lifters and bodybuilders in the Soviet Union and other Eastern bloc countries used steroids to improve their strength. The results spoke for themselves: In the 1952 Olympic Games, the Soviets won seven medals in the weight lifting events. Spectators were amazed at the strength of those athletes. The progress of the Soviets impressed one observer in particular, Dr. John Ziegler, who was a medical adviser for the U.S. Olympic team.

"They'd Have Eaten Rat Manure"

After speaking with a Soviet team physician and learning that the athletes were using testosterone, Ziegler was concerned. He worried that the Soviets were going to exploit their success at the Olympics politically—a valid concern, since sports at that time were often a proving ground between the superpowers during the cold war. "I felt the Russians were going to use sports as the biggest international publicity trick going . . . and strength sports especially," he later explained. "They saw it as a political advantage 100 percent."[3]

Not wanting the United States to fall behind in this arena, Ziegler went to an American pharmaceutical company with the idea of making the benefits of steroids available to U.S. athletes. The introduction of their product, called Dianabol, was eagerly received. Years later Ziegler admitted that American athletes would have tried anything to achieve the same results as their Soviet counterparts: "I honestly believe that if I'd told people back then that rat manure would make them stronger, they'd have eaten rat manure."[4]

"Players Sprinkled the Tablets on Their Cereal Like Sugar"

The results of the new drug were amazing; Dianabol was a favorite among weight lifters, bodybuilders, shot-putters, and discus throwers—and the list kept growing. Over the years, new kinds of steroids have been created, all of which seem to achieve the desired results, which has pleased athletes.

No one believed that there were harmful side effects associated with steroids at this time; it was completely legal for team doctors and trainers to prescribe steroids to athletes as a training tool. As they became more popular, athletes in other sports such as football and basketball began to use them, too.

Many athletes liked the results so much that they began increasing their dosages. Says Ziegler, "They figured if one pill was good, three or four would be better, and they were eating them like candy."[5] One former player in the National Football League (NFL) recalls that in the early 1960s, coaches and trainers placed bowls "heaped full of steroid tablets on dining tables, and players sprinkled the tablets on their cereal like sugar."[6]

Scary Side Effects

Partly because of such abuses of the drug, potential side effects were discovered in the 1960s. Users were likely to develop acne and experience balding. Steroids have also been linked to problems in the heart and lungs, increasing the risk of heart attack or stroke.

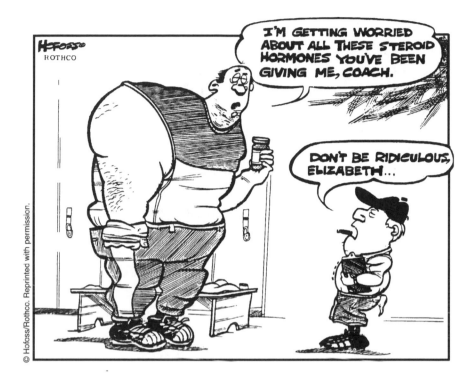

Liver abnormalities are another very serious risk. Some users have developed cancerous liver tumors; steroids can also cause blood-filled cysts to grow on the tissue of the liver.

Steroids have been found to cause problems in male and female reproductive systems, as well. Male users experience enlarged breasts, shrinkage of the testicles, and a lowering of the sperm count. In women, steroids cause a deep voice and increased body hair (especially on the face) and possible infertility or birth defects, should a woman user become pregnant.

Some disturbing psychological effects can occur from steroid use, too, such as bouts of uncontrolled aggression and hostility—for no apparent reason. Many users experience violent mood swings, going from lighthearted happiness to deep depression within a few moments. As one psychiatrist attests, "There are people with no history of violence or mood swings who will nevertheless go berserk on steroids, in rare cases becoming homicidal."[7]

Even So

By the late 1960s it was known that steroids used in large amounts could prove dangerous, and by the mid-1970s they joined stimulants and other harmful drugs on the Olympics' "banned" list.

Even though today doctors prescribe steroids for a number of legitimate medical purposes—for men whose natural hormone production is too low, or as a means of counteracting the effects of radiation in cancer treatment, for example—the sale or prescription of steroids as a performance enhancer for athletes is against the law in the United States.

Even so, there is a huge amount of trafficking of illegal steroids. Legally prescribed steroids account for a very small fraction of steroid drug use today. Legal sales account for about $3 million a year wholesale, while the black market in steroids—especially from Mexico, the primary source of illegal steroids—generates more than $780 million!

Hard to Resist

Why would athletes continue to take steroids, knowing that they are illegal, knowing that using them can result in serious health problems—even death? Quite simply, they work. They allow an athlete to get results from his or her body that just aren't possible without the drugs. As one doctor explains, "They can pump you up fast, increase your speed, decrease the time it takes to rebound from a serious workout, and often make you as ferocious as Mike Tyson with a bloodied nose."[8]

Harrison Pope, an associate doctor of psychiatry at Harvard, agrees wholeheartedly:

An athlete who is lackadaisical, who eats badly, sleeps badly, misses many days at the gym, works out without too much effort, and takes steroids can blow away an athlete who works out to the limit of his ability, sleeps perfectly, has a perfect diet, and in every other respect goes to the limit of his body.[9]

Pressures

Many experts say that another reason athletes are willing to risk their health on steroids is the enormous pressure to win. With the large salaries and signing bonuses for professional players, and the chance for even amateurs to make millions of dollars in endorsement fees, there is a great deal at stake in sports—on many levels, says one researcher:

> Victory brings increased status for the individual and his family, results in financial and career rewards, and boosts the image of the country. Defeat can result in personal humiliation, a loss of a career, and does nothing for the image of the athlete's country.[10]

If the athletes don't put enough pressure on themselves to excel, there are always coaches, trainers, even parents, who can subtly, or not so subtly, apply the pressure for a young person to do whatever it takes to win. One doctor confided, "I've gotten calls from parents wanting to know where to get steroids for their kids. One guy, calling about his seventh grade son, said he had all this potential to be an outstanding athlete, but just wasn't big enough."[11]

Testing as a Solution

How is the athletic community solving its drug problem? Testing is one way. In amateur athletics, such as collegiate events and the Olympics, athletes must have a sample of their urine tested for drugs before the results of a contest are official. If an athlete tests positive for a banned substance, as Canadian sprinter Ben Johnson did in the 1988 Olympic Games, he is stripped of his medal and banned from competition for a given length of time.

However, testing today is ineffective at best. Critics complain that the tests are too expensive and are not sensitive

enough to catch all chemical traces. There is also the danger
that a false positive can ruin an athlete's reputation—and in so
doing, detract from the sport itself. Insiders admit that there
have been more than a few athletes whose positive drug tests
were never revealed, simply because doing so would make
athletics look bad. The sports world, says one steroid expert,
"likes the benefits [of steroid use]. It gives world records,
bigger-than-life humans with tremendous physical capacities
they could not attain without drugs. That sells television commercials and endorsements."[12]

Others object to the idea of drug testing, complaining that
athletes are somehow being singled out as a group. They say
that athletes are merely a segment of a drug-using society—
no different from teachers, truck drivers, or CEOs. As one
writer argues:

> So why don't we test [Luciano] Pavarotti after every
> concert, or expunge Suede's albums from the charts if
> they were recorded while the artists were under the
> influence? . . . The music of Charlie Parker, a heroin
> addict, the acting of Cary Grant, who used LSD, the
> writing of Dylan Thomas, an alcoholic: all these have
> not been obliterated like Ben Johnson's [world record
> of] 9.79 seconds.[13]

Difficult Questions

The role of drugs in sports today poses some difficult questions that have prompted furious debate within the medical
and athletic communities. For example, while most doctors
agree that steroids pose definite health risks to users, they also
concede that little or no testing has been done on steroids that
can back up doctors' concerns.

Add to this the fact that steroid users often take the drugs
in dosages far exceeding those recommended and it's easy to
see why there is some degree of mystery. As one longtime
steroid advocate and author of a controversial booklet entitled

The Underground Steroid Handbook argues, "You cannot accept for a fact that steroids have harmful side effects. Some are more dangerous than others; some are not dangerous at all." [14]

There is also disagreement about whether certain performance-enhancing drugs should be banned at all. Some sports enthusiasts claim that athletes who use drugs to build muscle and increase endurance are cheating. Others, like one former Olympic coach, question why some advantages are labeled cheating and others not. One sports researcher noted that in a recent Olympic swimming competition, the American coach

> gleefully displayed a "greasy" swimsuit which allowed the women swimmers to improve upon their previous best times with the marginal advantage of reducing friction between the swimsuit and the water. He acknowledged that this small differential might well have been the difference between victory and defeat. [15]

Should sports be "pure" when society is not? Must they reflect society at all? Although no one can say how these issues will be resolved, it is clear that the way we as a society view athletes and athletics certainly lies in the balance.

1. Charlie Francis, *Speed Trap*. New York: St. Martin's Press, 1990.

2. Francis, *Speed Trap*.

3. Quoted in Bob Goldman and Ronald Klatz, *Death in the Locker Room: Drugs and Sports*. Chicago: Elite Sports Medicine Publications, 1992.

4. Quoted in Gary I. Wadler and Brian Hainline, *Drugs and the Athlete*. Philadelphia: F.A. Davis, 1989.

5. Quoted in Goldman and Klatz, *Death in the Locker Room*.

6. Quoted in Lisa Angowski Rogak, *Steroids: Dangerous Game*. Minneapolis: Lerner Publications, 1992.

7. Quoted in Skip Rozin, "Steroids: A Spreading Peril," *Business Week*, June 19, 1995.

8. Rozin, "Steroids: A Spreading Peril."

9. Quoted in Skip Rozin, "Steroids and Sports: What Price Glory?" *Business Week*, October 17, 1994.

10. Tom Donohoe and Neil Johnson, *Foul Play: Drug Abuse in Sports*. Oxford: Basil Blackwell, 1986.

11. Rozin, "Steroids: A Spreading Peril."

12. Quoted in Rozin, "Steroids: A Spreading Peril."

13. Ellis Cashmore, "Run of the Pill," *New Statesman and Society*, November 11, 1994.

14. Quoted in Don Nardo, *Drugs and Sports*. San Diego: Lucent Books, 1990.

15. Norman C. Fost, "Ethical and Social Issues in Antidoping Strategies in Sport," in *Sport . . . The Third Millennium/Sport . . . Le Troisieme Millenaire*, ed. Fernand Landry, Marc Landry, and Magdeleine Yerles. Quebec: Presses de L'Universite Laval, 1991.

CHAPTER 1

Is Drug Use a Serious Problem in Sports?

"The potential side effects of anabolic steroids were clearly very dangerous."

Steroids Are Life Threatening to Athletes

Jeff O'Brien, the last person in our town whose name you'd expect to see in the obituaries, was buried last Friday morning. He was only twenty-one years old—a clean-cut kid who just a few years back was captain of his high school football team. He had played some college ball, too, and had done well. At the time of his death, he had loving parents, two sisters, and too many friends to count.

Jeff didn't die from AIDS, a gang beating, or a car accident. He was not clinically depressed, and he did not die by his own hand. No, what killed him was drugs—although I bet he would have been astonished if anyone had identified the stuff he used as "hard drugs." Using anabolic steroids, chemicals he injected to gain strength and muscle mass, he suffered a massive, fatal heart attack. Yes, steroids killed Jeff O'Brien, and I am afraid that they are killing thousands of other young people like him.

Chemical Time Bombs

It's important to understand just what steroids are—and what they aren't. It is a fact, for instance, that not all steroids are potentially harmful. Doctors prescribe steroids for a number of legitimate reasons—certain eye diseases, intestinal disorders, arthritis, cancer, and asthma, for starters. Taken under a doctor's care, these steroids can bring relief from a host of debilitating health problems.

The culprits are those chemicals that are forms of testosterone, the male sex hormone that makes men stronger, leaner, and more muscular. These steroids are known as anabolic (tissue building) and androgenic (giving rise to masculine characteristics), or AAS. These compounds of male sex hormones, when injected or ingested, make athletes chemical time bombs.

From Nazi Troops to Athletes

This is not to say that the anabolic-androgenic steroids don't deliver on their promise of adding muscle mass, strength, and endurance. Scientists have been aware of these properties for decades. (AAS also produce heightened aggressiveness, which is why Hitler's armies were given the drugs during World War II.) The danger of AAS lies in the frightening side effects that are not included in the drug's claims.

Dr. Bob Goldman, investigating AAS in the 1970s after a friend developed what proved to be fatal kidney tumors from the steroids, found that medical journals cite a large number of other side effects. The literature, he writes,

> indicated that anabolic steroids could also inhibit growth in young athletes; cause high blood pressure, sterility, bleeding from the intestinal track, and hypoglycemia, increase the risk of heart attack, masculinize women, produce unsightly acne, deepen the voice, and change the distribution of body hair. The potential side effects of anabolic steroids were clearly very dangerous, and some were permanent.[1]

Doctors warn that it is chemically impossible for a steroid user to get the positive effects of the anabolic part of the drug without great risk from the androgenic part. Says one expert,

The Consequences of Steroid Use

Below is a listing of the various health problems and conditions caused by steroid use. These consequences have been grouped according to gender.

In males	In females
▶ impotence	▶ irreversible male-pattern baldness
▶ breast enlargement	▶ irreversible lowering of the voice
▶ sterility	▶ menstrual irregularities
▶ shrinking of the testicles	▶ decreased breast size
▶ enlargement of the prostate gland, which can lead to difficulty urinating	▶ irreversible and excessive hair growth on body

Source: National Association of State High School Associations.

"There isn't an anabolic-androgenic steroid an athlete can take to increase muscle mass, endurance, or speed, without risking dangerous hormonal side effects."[2]

"Walking, Talking Pharmacies"

Young athletes taking AAS—and recent studies estimate there could be as many as 750,000 teens on the drug—are especially vulnerable to the side effects, primarily because young people generally don't concern themselves with risk. One teen who has used AAS for three years admits he has experienced some of the unpleasant effects of the drug, but he isn't concerned. "I get side effects," he says, "like bloating, acne, and a sore chest and nipples. But I don't mind. It lets me know the stuff is working."[3]

The most frightening aspect of steroid use among athletes is that a great many of them are taking the drugs in dosages far exceeding what would be considered the "prescribed" dosage. Users commonly take AAS in cycles that last anywhere from four to eighteen weeks, followed by a long break. But many athletes panic during the break when some of the muscle and weight they've packed on with steroids diminishes. "Many panic," writes one researcher, "turning back to the drugs in even larger doses."[4]

And the dosages are staggering. Many physicians report that athletes are using one hundred to one thousand times the recommended dosage. Others are playing with dynamite, mixing and matching various brands of AAS—sometimes taking up to fourteen different drugs simultaneously in a process known as "stacking." As one teen remarked, "You wouldn't believe how much some guys go nuts on the stuff. They turn into walking, talking pharmacies."[5]

"You Couldn't Touch Me Because I Hurt So Much"

In an account of his steroid use as a fourteen-year-old, one young man explains his usage of a drug called Anatest, which is intended not for humans but for racehorses.

> The dosage was 1 cc (100 mg/cc) per ton of horse flesh. I didn't see the instructions, as a family member had given it to me. . . . The day after my first injection (enough for 1,200 lbs. of horse), I gained six pounds, and you couldn't touch me because I hurt so much. . . . Ultimately I gained 40 pounds of muscle in about a month.[6]

His second cycle was even more dangerous, he explains, because he changed to an oil-based steroid for which he had no instructions.

> I got a wicked GI [gastrointestinal] bleed from this . . . which nearly resulted in my death and *did* result in a one month hospitalization. The strength increases were astounding, but essentially useless when I couldn't even go to the bathroom on my own because I was hooked up to . . . life support systems.[7]

A Deadly List

This young man survived to tell about it, however, so we must consider him one of the lucky ones. Not so lucky are a long list of athletes—both amateur and professional—who died as a result of steroid use.

One well-known athlete was Lyle Alzado, who died of a brain tumor in 1992. Alzado, who had played for fourteen years in the NFL, was known for his muscular physique and his aggressive play. When doctors confirmed the presence of a cancerous brain tumor in 1991, Alzado explained that he had

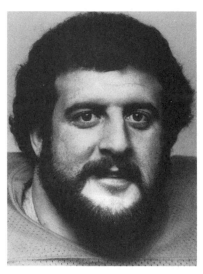

taken steroids and a dangerous steroid-related drug for twenty years, spending about $30,000 annually on them. Admitted Alzado, "I lied to a lot of people for a lot of years when I said I didn't use steroids."[8]

The brain tumor killed Alzado, but other chilling side effects from the steroid alternative he took were lurking just around the corner. That particular drug, used by doctors to treat dwarfism by stimulating growth, has been linked

Lyle Alzado

to acromegaly, or "Frankenstein's syndrome." This condition leads to distortion of the face, feet, and hands—before eventually killing its victims.

Not Exceptions

It's so important to get the message out to athletes—especially the young ones—that Lyle Alzado and Jeff O'Brien are not exceptions. Every week in clinics all across America, doctors are seeing the signs of steroid use and abuse. They are forced to tell athletes—from the teenage football hopefuls to the twenty-five-year-old professional bodybuilders—about a mass on a kidney, or a suspicious-sounding noise in their lungs.

It's time to get the message out loud and clear: The benefits of a chemically built body can't begin to outweigh the risks. Athletes should stay far away from anabolic-androgenic steroids.

1. Bob Goldman and Ronald Klatz, *Death in the Locker Room: Drugs and Sports*. Chicago: Elite Sports Medicine Publications, 1992.

2. Robert Voy, *Drugs, Sport, and Politics*. Champaign, IL: Leisure Press, 1991.

3. Quoted in Joannie M. Schrof, "Pumped Up," *U.S. News & World Report*, June 1, 1992.

4. Schrof, "Pumped Up."

5. Quoted in Schrof, "Pumped Up."

6. "The First and Only Time I Used Steroids," winning contest entry, Belle International, November 1997.

7. "The First and Only Time."

8. Quoted in Hank Nuwer, *Sports Scandals*. New York: Franklin Watts, 1994.

"For many athletes, these 'psychotic behaviors' were part of the allure of steroids."

Steroids Cause Serious Psychological Problems for Athletes

In 1988 Harvard psychologist Harrison Pope Jr. and his associate, David Katz, published the results of their research on forty-one athletes who were heavy steroid users. It was found that 12 percent of them had suffered psychotic symptoms while using the drugs—from aggression and profound depression to delusions and paranoia. In addition, 30 percent of them acknowledged that they experienced mood swings while on steroids.

Psychotic behavior while on steroids? Though perhaps causing a stir within the scientific community, athletes were not even mildly interested. "It was like finding out that not brushing your teeth causes cavities," shrugs one bodybuilder. "Everybody knew that already."[1]

'Roid Rage

For many athletes, these "psychotic behaviors" were part of the allure of steroids in the first place. Many football players, for example, would consider the explosive aggressiveness (a common side effect of steroid use) a very positive, admirable quality. One college football player who took steroids reported later that he loved the feeling of being a loose cannon, because he played with more energy. Those feelings continued throughout the day; he reportedly needed only two or three hours of sleep each night, and he would wake up, in his words, "indestructible, angry, and ready to kick butt." He explained to one college sports reporter after he stopped using steroids that the drug he was taking "changes you; it makes you an ego monster."[2]

Although the increased aggression would please their coaches and teammates, some users found that more and more often they were "crossing the line" in their play—from aggression to violence. One former steroid user recalls wanting to do permanent harm to the running back he was tackling, looking for ways to make cheap shots without getting called on it by game officials.

Other steroid users found that "'roid rage," as it has been termed, began to have an effect on their personal relationships, too. "The athlete cannot turn these [aggressive] feelings off once the competition is over," says one doctor. "I have heard from girlfriends and wives of AAS users the fears that they have when their boyfriends and spouses are 'cycling' on these drugs."[3]

Dr. Jekyll and Mr. Hyde

One of the most upsetting aspects of 'roid rage is the suddenness of it, say experts. "There doesn't appear to be a limit to the amount an individual might change," comments Robert Voy, who has served as the chief medical officer for the U.S. Olympic Committee. "This syndrome closely resembles the classic Dr. Jekyll and Mr. Hyde personality."[4] The parents of one eighteen-year-old user claim that they could never predict when their son's rage would surface. "Once, he pounded dents into the hood of the family car. He alternated between rational and irrational thoughts. . . . Once, when someone cut him off, [he] pulled the man over and beat him up."[5]

Reports of such incidents are almost too numerous to count. A bodybuilder on steroids attacks a stranger with a crowbar after a minor accident in a parking lot. A normally pleasant teen throws his full dinner plate at his father when he refuses to loan the boy $50. And it isn't limited to male users, either. Tina Plakinger, a former women's national bodybuilding champion, claimed that the drugs she was taking made her so angry that she grabbed her husband and forced him up against the wall one night—for being twenty minutes late for dinner!

Too Much Testosterone

Doctors know that testosterone can induce aggression and violence in other animals, so it should not be much of a surprise when the same results occur in humans. The treatment of hens with synthetic testosterone, for instance, has been shown to induce enough "henpecking" and aggression that the social order of the flock is disrupted. In rats, too, injections of anabolic steroids caused overaggressive behavior among both sexes, and greatly increased the intensity of fighting that male rats engaged in.

Because of the hormonal shifting that is normal for their age, teenagers often experience mood swings and irritability. So are we shocked when steroids produce the same results, and more? As one researcher says, "If natural biological changes [in teens] can cause such marked shifts of mood, how much more dramatic must they be in someone who is ingesting or injecting very high doses of male sex hormones?"[6]

We as a society are already painfully aware of how certain recreational drugs can create monsters. PCP, crack, speed—the newspapers are filled with horror stories about criminals acting under their influence.

"I told myself for a year and a half that I had to get off steroids," says one former user. "I kept lying to my girlfriend, always reassuring her nothing was wrong. But she noticed, man. And when she was noticing too much and it bugged me, I'd lash out. One time I almost busted her jaw. I can't think about those days without feeling real ashamed."[7]

Just because steroids are taken in well-lit gyms instead of back alleys doesn't make them less threatening.

1. Dana, interview with author, Minneapolis, MN, December 1, 1997.

2. Quoted in "IOC Removes Seven Drug-Testing Labs from Its Approved List," *NCAA News*, April 12, 1989.

3. Robert Voy, *Drugs, Sport, and Politics*. Champaign, IL: Leisure Press, 1991.

4. Voy, *Drugs*.

5. Quoted in William N. Taylor, *Macho Medicine: A History of the Anabolic Steroid Epidemic*. Jefferson, NC: McFarland, 1991.

6. James E. Wright and Virginia S. Cowart, *Anabolic Steroids: Altered States*. Carmel, IN: Benchmark Press, 1990.

7. Dana, personal interview.

"Anyone taking steroids is at risk, but teenagers are especially vulnerable."

Steroids Present a Growing Danger to Teen Athletes

One would be hard-pressed these days to name a professional sport that has not been tainted by the stain of drug abuse. In fact, one could almost name a player on every pro team—whether hockey, basketball, football, or baseball—who has made headlines not because of outstanding play but because of drug use and the consequent trouble it has caused. Such an exercise would be a reminder that our sports heroes are not always the role models we'd like them to be—and that would be somewhat disappointing, I'll admit.

But what really saddens me is not that the tiny slice of the nation's athletes that we watch on television have a drug problem. Rather, it's the fact that there are a staggering number of athletes whose names will never be known (at least above the high school level) who are swallowing or injecting every drug in the book that they believe can give them at least a chance to be like those million-dollar sports stars on television. I'm frightened for our teenage athletes—boys and girls—who are chemically altering their bodies by the tens of thousands every day.

Steroids, the Biggest Problem

By far, the biggest drug threat to teens today is anabolic steroids—the supersized doses of the male hormone testosterone that can give young athletes heftier builds, faster legs, and better endurance. While perhaps in the old days kids would train for their chosen sport by lifting weights and running, today's athletes know that they don't need to work out with the same intensity. There are shortcuts, and teenagers are taking them in astonishingly high numbers.

Researchers at Pennsylvania State University estimated in 1987 that as many as 500,000 teenage boys were using steroids; however, ten years later, experts say that the 1987 figure has probably tripled. The Illinois Department of Alcohol and Substance Abuse found that between 7 and 11 percent of teenagers have at least experimented with such drugs, and that teenage girls are now the fastest-growing user group.

"Everybody wants to get big, that's all," says one seventeen-year-old steroid user.

> I know girls who are using not to look all big like guys, but to get the legs and speed for track and basketball. It's not that rare anymore. The boys start 'cause you see these guys who use and they are everything you want to be. When you're skinny and small and 13, 14 years old, you figure you don't have much to lose, and everything to gain.[1]

Another young user agrees. "Our role model is this older guy, the biggest guy at the gym. He's not a nice guy, but he weighs 290 pounds without an ounce of fat . . . that's our goal."[2]

More Risks for Teens

Of course, there are lots of dangers when you begin to dabble in drugs like steroids. The serious side effects of the drug, such as liver tumors and heart problems, are well documented. So are the shrinking of the testicles and the formation of breasts in males, and the deepening of the voice and the appearance of hair on the face and body in females.

Anyone taking steroids is at risk, but teenagers are especially vulnerable. Acknowledges one chemical dependency counselor, "Even a brief period of abuse could have lasting effects on a child whose body and brain chemistry are still developing."[3]

Ironically, teenage athletes who use steroids to increase their size often end up with smaller bodies than they would have had they not taken the drugs. Researchers know that the growth plates on the ends of bones close prematurely, so a steroid user's adult height is shorter than it would have been. Teenage girls who use steroids are facing the cessation of menstrual periods and are putting their reproductive systems in jeopardy.

Who's to Blame?

What's going on here? Hundreds of thousands of teens are permanently damaging their bodies—and facing death—by using steroids. Aren't we getting the antisteroid message out, as we do for cigarettes, marijuana, and cocaine?

Surprisingly, kids *are* being educated about the dangers of steroids, but all that education is having a less than desirable effect—at times even backfiring. A statewide steroid-education program in Oregon, for example, resulted in students who were statistically more likely to use steroids "even if it caused a 50 percent risk of dying within 20 to 30 years."[4]

Many experts place the blame on the importance we as a society place on physical beauty. "The way society—in particular, the opposite sex—views our physical attractiveness," declares one nationally recognized bodybuilder, "probably contributes more to our self-image concept than does any other factor, especially in teenagers. . . . Our society thrives on physical excellence. It has become an American value."[5]

Others point to teenagers' feelings of invincibility as the cause, saying that young people tend to place more importance on short-range effects than on long-range ones. For example, one poll of teen steroid users found that 82 percent said they didn't believe that steroids were harming them much, and, even more striking, 40 percent said they wouldn't stop, even if they thought they were being harmed.

Winning Is the Only Thing

Other studies seem to bear this out. A recent survey of high school track athletes asked participants to consider the following dilemma: You can take a drug that is illegal and possibly dangerous to your health, but it will make you an Olympic-level runner. Would you take the drug? More than 80 percent said yes—without question.

The results are a frightening picture of what our society is saying about sports today. In years gone by, parents would tell their children, "Winning isn't everything." Today the advice is more like that of the legendary Green Bay Packers coach Vince Lombardi: "Winning isn't everything—it's the only thing."

What we are telling our children, our teenage athletes— and what we are allowing their coaches to tell them—is that we are not happy with them merely participating in sports. There is no value inherent in athletics; successful results are

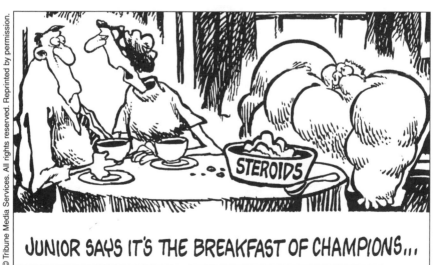

JUNIOR SAYS IT'S THE BREAKFAST OF CHAMPIONS...

all that matters. As one steroid expert explains, "We don't allow our kids to play games for fun anymore. We preach that God really does win on Friday night, when we should be teaching our children to be satisfied to finish 27th, if that's their personal best."[6]

It's time we recognized that teens are at an extremely fragile time in their lives, both physically and emotionally. We need to remind them that the use of steroids to improve athletic prowess is not a healthy way to live their lives. Not even if they win the state title or have college scouts panting after them. Not ever, because it isn't worth the risk. No game ever is.

1. Pete, interview with author, Bloomington, MN, December 9, 1997.

2. Quoted in Joannie M. Schrof, "Pumped Up," *U.S. News & World Report*, June 1, 1992.

3. Quoted in Schrof, "Pumped Up."

4. James E. Wright and Virginia S. Cowart, *Anabolic Steroids: Altered States*. Carmel, IN: Benchmark Press, 1990.

5. Sergio Oliveira, "The Steroid Problem: 'Roid Truth from a Man Who Knows," *Musclemag*, September 1995.

6. Quoted in Schrof, "Pumped Up."

"Not only are steroids not a great danger, they are actually a harmless tool in the hands of serious athletes."

The Danger of Steroids Is Exaggerated

We've all heard the horrible stories—tales of kids too young to shave who are going bald and becoming sterile from using steroids. And stories of the girls who *need* to shave, whose voices deepen while their breasts shrink. And those aren't even the scariest parts. No, what the really awful effects of steroids are can't even be noticed from the outside—the weakening of the heart and lungs, the craziness that happens in the brain, the cancer that blooms in the liver.

Media Hype

We're clearly meant to be frightened by these stories, and as a result, to shun the use of steroids—in the same manner, for instance, as we are to shun the use of cigars and cigarettes. The problem is that while the hazards of smoking tobacco are well documented and medically sound, the data on steroids is confusing and, at the very least, inconclusive. Even so, the media have seized on certain supposed "steroid deaths" as a way of scaring young athletes away from steroids. But the media's message is flawed, because it is not accurate.

Take the well-known case of NFL star Lyle Alzado, who died of a brain tumor he announced was the result of taking steroids. Alzado's death is often mentioned as one of the "tragedies" of steroid use. But let's keep in mind that Alzado, by his own admission, had taken steroids for twenty years, as, he claimed, most other NFL players had. From two decades of heavy steroid use, he had suffered no ill effects.

No Proof

Then he decides to make a comeback into professional football and used something called human growth hormone, which is *not* a steroid. He then developed a cancerous brain tumor, which in time killed him. The question seems obvious: How do we know what caused the brain tumor that killed Alzado?

The answer is, We don't know. We don't have a clue, because, as one steroid expert says, "No evidence was produced to support Alzado's claim, and no controlled studies or research have ever shown that steroids can produce such a neurological possibility."[1]

In other words, all that doctors know is that a tumor killed Lyle Alzado. No one can say what caused the tumor. He might have contracted a tumor through his genetic makeup, or from pollutants, or whatever it is that non–steroid users who contract brain tumors get them from.

Before we jump on the antisteroid bandwagon, doesn't it seem intelligent to at least get the facts? Before we condemn these drugs, one expert writes, "either long-term prospective studies are needed, or at least better retrospective case control studies with careful design and analysis by expert epidemiologists."[2]

'Roid Rage?

Another of the supposed ill effects of steroids is the phenomenon known as 'roid rage, a kind of psychotic behavior that exhibits itself in the form of uncontrollable anger, sometimes followed by deep depression. This alleged side effect of steroid use has been repeated so often, we must remind ourselves that there has been absolutely no clinical study that has shown it even exists.

On the contrary, in a recent study reported in the *New England Journal of Medicine*, biologist Shalender Bhasin and his colleagues found that "the psychological condition known as 'roid rage was largely a myth . . . [and that] moderate doses . . . are relatively safe."[3] No anger, no behavioral abnormalities, nothing.

Although NFL star Lyle Alzado believed his long-term steroid use caused his fatal brain tumor, no evidence was found to support his claim.

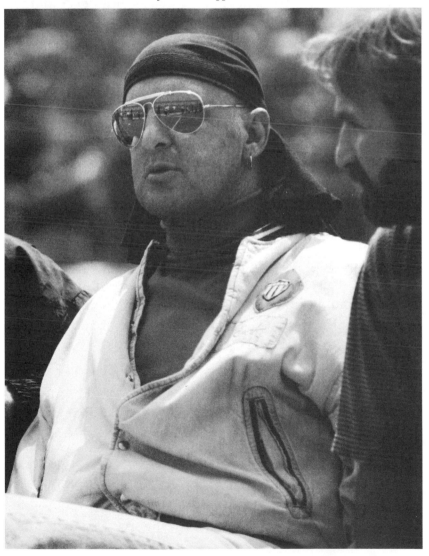

It is true, of course, that many users "stack" various steroids, using very large doses that surpass those used in the Bhasin study. One example is bodybuilder Sergio Oliveira, who admits to using steroids continuously for eight years "in dosages that would absolutely horrify the worst of steroid users, often having testosterone levels that would exceed those of a pack of large, male gorillas."[4] Oliveira is bemused by all the talk of 'roid rage and other steroid dangers among athletes, saying that these side effects "are just not developing in the bodybuilders and athletes who have been using steroids for over three decades."[5]

"It's Not for Everyone"

Some would push the argument a bit further, saying that not only are steroids *not* a great danger, they are actually a harmless tool in the hands of serious athletes. One such advocate is Daniel Duchaine, whose *Underground Steroid Handbook* is a widely distributed guide for the users of steroids and other performance-enhancing drugs. Duchaine does not promote the use of drugs for young people but feels strongly that steroid use has proven beneficial to his overall well-being, and he scoffs at the warnings that so-called medical experts give about the drugs. "I know that proper steroid therapy can enhance your health," he claims in his handbook. "Do you believe someone just because he has an M.D. or a Ph.D. stuck onto the end of his name?"[6]

Other users agree:

> I don't want to tell anyone else what to do, because if someone was [telling] me, I wouldn't listen, I guess. It's not for everyone. But I'm a living, breathing user of steroids. I don't have female breasts, I'm not losing my hair, and I haven't got liver cancer or anything like that. What I do have is a great body, and I'm stronger than any of my brothers. I like how I look, and I work hard [in the gym] to maintain it.[7]

Abuse Is the Problem

This doesn't mean that there aren't potential problems. Like any drug, steroids can be misused—or overused. That can be said of penicillin or aspirin, too. But such potential for abuse is not a reason to ban a drug.

If society is squeamish about the use of steroids and any other performance-enhancing drugs in sports, let's discuss that as an ethical issue, one of fair play. But let's not pretend, as the medical community has done in the past, that there is evidence that steroids are life-threatening. As even Penn State University's Charles Yesalis—who is definitely on the side of banning the use of steroids—admits, "This doesn't appear to be a killer drug. Don't quote me as saying they're good for you or harmless, but I can't give you more than a handful of steroid deaths."[8]

This surely doesn't sound like any reason to sound the alarms, does it?

1. Sergio Oliveira, "The Steroid Problem: 'Roid Truth from a Man Who Knows," *Musclemag*, September 1995.

2. Norman C. Fost, "Ethical and Social Issues in Antidoping Strategies in Sport," in *Sport . . . the Third Millennium/Sport . . . Le Troisieme Millenaire*, ed. Fernand Landry, Marc Landry, and Magdeleine Yerles. Quebec: Presses de L'Universite Laval, 1991.

3. Quoted in Jose Antonio, "What the Media Missed on 'Roid Rage," *Muscle & Fitness*, January 1997.

4. Oliveira, "The Steroid Problem."

5. Oliveira, "The Steroid Problem."

6. Quoted in Joannie M. Schrof, "Pumped Up," *U.S. News & World Report*, June 1, 1992.

7. Interview with author (name withheld by request), December 13, 1997.

8. Quoted in Skip Rozin, "Steroids and Sports: What Price Glory?" *Business Week*, October 17, 1994.

CHAPTER 2

Why Do Athletes Take Drugs?

*"It is the people in whom young athletes put their trust—
their coaches and trainers—who are pressuring them to
use drugs."*

Coaches and Team Doctors Encourage Athlete Drug Use

There are many aspects of the link between sports and drugs that are shameful. It is shameful, for instance, that so many young athletes are willing to inject and ingest chemicals into their bodies when those chemicals might be harmful—even lethal. It is shameful that the idea of fair play and sportsmanship has eroded to the extent that athletes must be tested for chemicals that give them unfair advantages.

But nothing is as sad as the fact that it is the people in whom young athletes put their trust—their coaches and trainers—who are pressuring them to use drugs to enhance their performance. So prevalent is the breach of trust, reports a 1992 survey by the Illinois Department of Alcoholism and Substance Abuse, that 21 percent of high school athletes using steroids admit that their supplier was a coach or teacher.

Kinds of Pressure

The pressure coaches apply toward their athletes can take various forms. Some are vague hints—"We sure need you as linebacker next year, John, but you've got to find a way to pack on

41

some muscle pretty quick," for instance. Others, like the one
East German sprinter Renate Neufield received from her
coaches, are more obvious.

In December 1978, Neufield revealed that she had been
forced by her coaches to take steroids. Reports one source:

> She experienced a range of unpleasant side effects
> including abnormal hair growth and menstrual dis-
> turbances. When she refused to take the drugs,
> Neufield claimed she was interrogated, and alleged
> that there were threats of reprisal aimed at her and
> her family. Neufield defected to the West in 1977 after
> the "psychological pressure" became too intense.[1]

"I Was Approached on Numerous Occasions"

Sound far-fetched? Or maybe something that could only happen in some of those Eastern European countries where
strategies for winning Olympic events are supposedly planned
out as carefully as any war?

Unfortunately for the world of sports—and for a great
many young athletes today—this is not far-fetched at all. And
coaches in the United States, unfortunately, are some of the
worst offenders. Take Chuck DeBus, a track and field coach
from Santa Monica, California. According to Dr. Robert Voy,
former chief medical officer for the U.S. Olympic Committee, DeBus "has built a reputation for sending this message to
many of his athletes: If you don't want to use drugs, I don't
want to work with you."[2]

U.S. javelin thrower Marilyn White attests to this assessment of her former coach. "I was approached on numerous
occasions by . . . DeBus to begin a training program that included the daily use of steroids. . . . Mr. DeBus stated that I
would never be good enough to become a national contender
unless I were to take steroids."[3]

Easy Motivation

It's certainly not difficult to understand the motivation of
coaches who push dangerous drugs onto the athletes under

their guidance. After all, steroids create players who can run faster, throw farther, or tackle harder. And players like that win—pure and simple. As steroid expert Charles Yesalis notes: "Sports likes the benefits of steroids. It gives world records, bigger-than-life humans with tremendous physical capacities that sell television minutes and fill stadiums."[4]

But what about the health of the athlete? Don't coaches and trainers worry that the drugs they are pushing today may result in serious health concerns later in life?

The answer is a resounding "no." Coaches and trainers, say experts, are not concerned with anything more remote than the next race or the next big game. As one doctor who asked to remain anonymous explains:

> As a generality, team physicians tend to be men of action, not scholarly, speculative types. They are interested in immediate problems, making somebody strong, relaxed, mean, or quick, and in getting a player back in the game as soon as possible. If somebody tells them there is a drug that might do the trick, they are apt to try it. They are not likely to wait for a double-blind control study to find out if the drug is effective or what it will do to the liver three years later. They are interested in today.[5]

Pieces of Meat?

Others in the medical profession agree. "We are . . . a highly competitive society," says one drug researcher, "where a win-at-any-cost philosophy prevails. Quite simply, also-rans [contestants who do not win], regardless of their effort, are rewarded disproportionately, if at all."[6]

Such attitudes dehumanize individual players and make it easy for coaches to treat players as if they were mere chattel, pieces of meat. The trick, it seems, is to use a player until he no longer has anything to offer. Then, because he is expendable, he can be replaced by a fresh face and a healthy body.

Take the example of former Chicago Bears lineman Dick Butkus. The last years of his career he had been plagued by aching, swollen knees. Rather than allow him to rest (the usual treatment), team doctor Theodore Fox repeatedly shot his knees full of cortisone and other drugs to deaden the pain, making it possible for him to play. Butkus later sued the doc-

Former Chicago Bears lineman Dick Butkus sued team doctor Theodore Fox for injecting cortisone and other painkillers into Butkus's injured knees instead of demanding he stay off his legs. The judge sided with Butkus in the lawsuit.

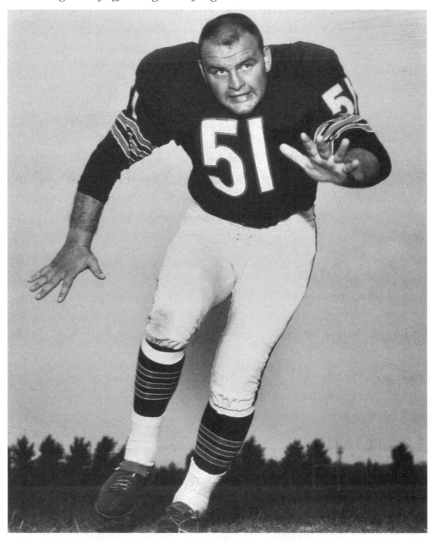

tor, and the court sided with Butkus. "What Butkus was alleging," reports sportswriter Joseph Nocera, "was that . . . Fox had put the short-term needs of the team over Butkus's long-term health."[7]

Just four years later, NBA center Bill Walton made a similar charge against the team physician for the Portland Trail Blazers, Robert Cook. Walton claimed that Cook had done permanent injury to him by numbing his feet with painkillers before each game. Like Butkus's lawsuit, this case was settled in Walton's favor. And like Butkus's lawsuit, Walton's clearly showed the American public how professional teams (in football and basketball, at least) encourage the use of drugs for their players—not to heal, but to extend the use of that player for one more game, one more championship. The health of the player is irrelevant, it seems.

Without question, our society *is* cockeyed where sports are concerned. And undeniably the money and glamour of being a success are prizes too tempting for some people to use good judgment. But if the athletes themselves are at risk, if their health is compromised in the pursuit of Super Bowls or Olympic medals by those who work most closely with them, what sort of victories are these? And how can we as spectators cheer?

1. Tom Donohoe and Neil Johnson, *Foul Play: Drug Abuse in Sports*. Oxford: Basil Blackwell, 1986.

2. Robert Voy, *Drugs, Sport, and Politics*. Champaign, IL: Leisure Press, 1991.

3. Quoted in Voy, *Drugs, Sport, and Politics*.

4. Quoted in Skip Rozin, "Steroids and Sports: What Price Glory?" *Business Week*, October 17, 1994.

5. Quoted in Bob Goldman and Ronald Klatz, *Death in the Locker Room: Drugs and Sports*. Chicago: Elite Sports Medicine Publications, 1992.

6. Quoted in Hank Nuwer, *Steroids*. New York: Franklin Watts, 1990.

7. Joseph Nocera, "Bitter Medicine," *Sports Illustrated*, November 6, 1995.

"Young athletes are impressionable and eager to try something daring."

Immaturity Causes Athlete Drug Use

Canadian runner Ben Johnson had never looked as powerful and strong as he did that September in Seoul, South Korea. It was the 100-meter dash, the event he knew he could win against an old rival, American Carl Lewis. Johnson's confidence was warranted—he not only beat Lewis but set a new world record of 9.79 seconds.

But the event proved disastrous for Johnson. A postevent drug test, in which he was required to have a sample of his urine tested for prohibited drugs, was positive. Johnson's gold medal was stripped from him, as he admitted to having used anabolic steroids for the past eight years.

The sporting public was aghast. Paul Dupre, president of Canada's track and field governing body, called the affair "a tragic embarrassment to the world amateur sport movement and to Canada."[1] Sportswriters were quick to blame his coach, his trainer, even society in general for making him do such a thing.

Johnson, who had come to Seoul after running blistering races in various international competitions, found that he would lose more than his gold medal, however. His earlier successes had earned him more than $1 million in annual endorsements with companies like American Express Canada and

Mazda, but after his Olympic performance, those companies couldn't wait to distance themselves from him.

"This Former Athlete . . . Must Assume the Burden"

Johnson was given a two-year suspension from competing, and he vowed he would be back as a contender—without the drugs. "Whatever I lost doesn't mean a thing," he emphasized after the suspension was lifted. "I want to have children, get married. If I had kept taking [steroids], I could have side effects with my liver. I'm very glad I got caught."[2]

The Ben Johnson story might have had a happy ending if he had believed those words. However, whatever good intentions Johnson might have had in that 1990 interview disappeared by 1993. It was then that he received a lifetime ban from competition after testing positive for steroids again. This time there were no words of hope for his redemption, no laying of blame anywhere but where it truly belonged—squarely at the Adidas-clad feet of Ben Johnson himself. "This former athlete, alone," said Dupre, "must assume the burden of this latest embarrassment."[3]

It was, as sports agent Joe Douglas explains it, yet another case of an immature young athlete being incapable of thinking straight. He had had a taste of what "success" means in sports. And having lost it in 1988, Johnson found that coming back without steroids was not going to be easy. "All of a sudden there's attention, there's fame, there's money," says Douglas. "When you lose everything, I don't think anybody should be surprised that there's temptation."[4]

"Steroid McDonald's"

The temptation appears to be too much for a growing number of athletes. The use of drugs seems to be their way of dealing with a domain that measures success by having a shoe named after you in addition to a seven-figure salary for competing. There is no question that the riches to be reaped are

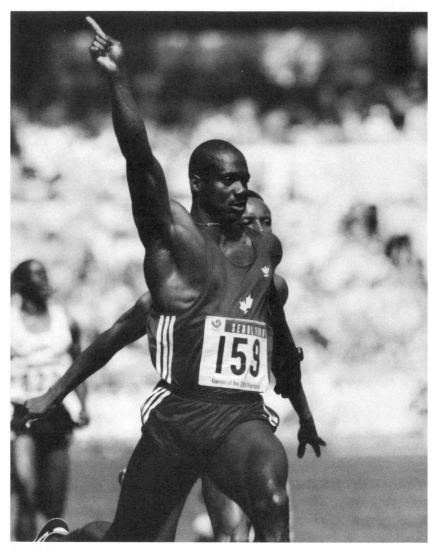

Ben Johnson set a new world record of 9.79 seconds in the 100-meter race in the 1988 Olympics in Seoul, South Korea. He was later stripped of his gold medal and banned from the sport for life after testing positive for steroids.

staggering. So, it seems, are the opportunities for these young, immature athletes to fall flat on their faces, so to speak.

One big indicator of this immaturity is evident in their reluctance to work hard for goals that may take years to attain. It's as though we've raised a whole new generation of kids who can't sit through anything longer than a sound bite.

When training and hard work are required, many athletes get restless. This is undoubtedly one of the main reasons steroid use is so popular. As one former trainer explains, "They [young steroid users] come from a gym environment, where muscle mentality pervades and creates a demand for bigger bench-presses, bigger squats. But they would rather not take a long-term approach. They want steroid McDonald's."[5]

Unconcerned with Health Issues

Another sure sign of their immaturity is the sense of invincibility they have about themselves. It's one of the things adults forget about the minute they start being adults: Young people don't think about getting hurt. In fact, that's more than likely a reason the best athletes play with such abandon. They aren't thinking about spraining muscles or twisting ankles. And they sure aren't thinking about the scary things drugs can do to their bodies.

"They [young athletes] don't see professional athletes dying from using steroids, but they do see them as being everything they want to be," explains one steroid expert. "They are the physically elite—big, strong, and fast. They are also popular, successful, attract beautiful women, and make lots of money. Why wouldn't [they] want to use steroids?"[6]

A European Olympic runner emphatically agrees. He sees many of his peers using a new "designer" drug that has already killed more than twenty-five athletes and can't believe that athletes are still eager to use it. "You have guys who will go to the funeral of a friend who died from this stuff," he says, "come home, and inject it again."[7]

Drug Dealers by the Locker-Room Door

Youth and immaturity are responsible for more than just steroid use, however. Over the years, cocaine—because of its high cost—has become the signature drug for the highly paid (and equally immature) professional athlete. Taken either to get a quick, euphoric high, as a way of masking the athlete's chronic aches and pains, or to provoke aggressiveness before a big game, coke is all too common in and around locker rooms today.

Part of the reason for its popularity, say experts, is that young athletes are impressionable and eager to try something daring. In his early days as a team physician for college football players, Robert Voy remembers cocaine pushers regularly approaching up-and-coming athletes.

> It was interesting to see drug dealers waiting at airports or outside locker room entrances to actually stuff pouches of cocaine into the gym bags of athletes passing by. Giving an athlete a few grams of coke on the house seemed like an investment to them. Once the pusher hooked a topflight athlete, he . . . had a prime customer.[8]

Why play around with a drug that can prove addictive the first time one uses it? Again, immaturity—that "It won't happen to me" attitude that doesn't seem to pay off real well. All a young phenom with pockets full of money needs to do is scan the sports pages (which read more and more like a police blotter these days) and see the bad things that "didn't happen" to other phenoms.

"He Was So Cool, He's Cold"

Read about the Dwight Goodens, the Mercury Morrises, the "Hollywood" Hendersons. Read about Len Bias, the basketball superstar who had it made the night he was drafted the number one pick by the Boston Celtics, until he decided to do a little coke with a few of his teammates. A few hours later he was on a slab in the mortuary.

Some college coaches who had seen Bias play were saddened by the incident, but many were disgusted by the immaturity that led to an unnecessary death. Indiana coach Bobby Knight reacted this way:

I don't feel sorry for Len Bias. Len Bias had his own mind and his own body to take care of, and he didn't do it. . . . Len Bias was better than anybody in this room . . . but he's dead. He's not sick, he's not hurt, he's dead. He just wasn't strong enough to take care of himself. He wanted to be one of the boys. He wanted to be cool. Well, he was so cool, he's cold. He's as cold as heck.[9]

Former Maryland forward Len Bias dunks the ball at a game against Miami University of Ohio. The same night that Bias was drafted as the first pick by the Boston Celtics, he died of a cocaine overdose.

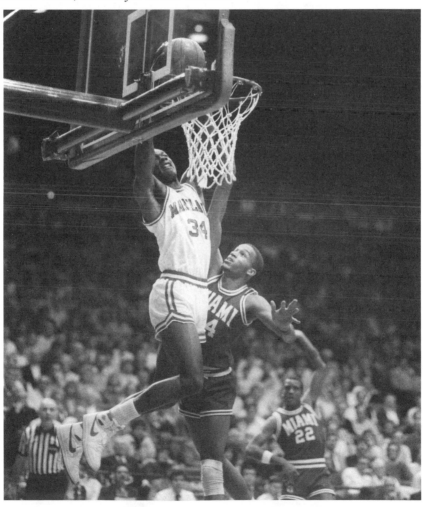

"An Exciting Way to Escape"

Psychologists who have worked with professional athletes know that much of their drug trouble begins with their inexperience in handling all the responsibilities of the job. As one writer observed:

> There's all that money. There's all that fame. There's all that public adulation. And there are all those constant demands made on you by the team, by the fans, and by yourself. Win. Outperform your opponent so that your salary is justified and your pride maintained. Never let down—because if you do, there's always someone waiting to step in and take over your job.[10]

Little wonder that many young athletes are taking refuge in drugs—whether to bulk up and maintain their edge or as a release from the daily pressures. Major League Baseball player Darryl Strawberry claims the drugs and bad living became a regular lifestyle for him. "Drink, do coke, get women, do something freaky," he says. "I played games when I was drunk, or just getting off a drunk or all night partying or coming down [from] amphetamines. . . . It was an exciting way to escape from everything else."[11]

It's a seamy side of athletics. We have young kids who can shoot a basketball or run a one-hundred-meter race or run back a punt, but they haven't got a clue how to manage themselves. We give them megasalaries, lots of time on their hands, and hope for the best. Certainly a surefire recipe for disaster. But then, what did we expect?

1. Quoted in Mary Nemeth, "Scandal: Act 2," *MacLean's*, March 15, 1993.

2. Quoted in Hank Nuwer, *Sports Scandals*. New York: Franklin Watts, 1994.

3. Quoted in Nemeth, "Scandal."

4. Quoted in Nemeth, "Scandal."

5. Quoted in Nuwer, *Sports Scandals*.

6. Sergio Oliveira, "The Steroid Problem: 'Roid Truth from a Man Who Knows," *Musclemag*, September 1995.

7. Quoted in Michael Bamberger and Don Yaeger, "Over the Edge," *Sports Illustrated*, April 14, 1997.

8. Robert Voy, *Drugs, Sport, and Politics*. Champaign, IL: Leisure Press, 1991.

9. Quoted in Mark Sabljak and Martin H. Greenberg, *Sports Babylon: Sex, Drugs, and Other Dirty Dealings in the World of Sports*. New York: Bell Publishing, 1988.

10. Edward F. Dolan, *Drugs in Sports*. New York: Franklin Watts, 1986.

11. Quoted in Tom Verducci, "The High Price of Hard Living," *Sports Illustrated*, February 27, 1995.

"There may be some athletes who can win gold medals without taking drugs, but they are few in number."

Athletes Take Drugs to Remain Competitive

There are lots of good arguments, both pro and con, about the use of steroids in sports. Some cite the much-publicized health risks—everything from cancer to kidney and liver problems to baldness and male breast growth—as reasons to ban the drugs. Others make a reasonable case that the use of performance-altering drugs is unethical, and therefore athletes who continue to use them are damaging the reputation of sports, both professional and amateur.

On the flip side, those who would like to see the ban on steroid use lifted point to the difficulty and unreliability of drug testing. Others find it a blurry line between substances such as steroids and other drugs that do not happen to be banned. Still others wonder about the accuracy of the health-risk reports of steroids, and even if they are dangerous, whether it is the job of the NFL, Major League Baseball, or the International Olympic Committee (to name but a few) to protect athletes from that danger.

Big Business, High Stakes

In a perfect world, perhaps, we could have an easy-to-administer drug test that would be so sensitive it could pick up *any* chem-

ical that has no business floating around in an athlete's blood-
stream. Or, if chemicals were to be allowed, we would modify
them so they were completely safe for the user. (Of course, in
a perfect world, athletes would be competing for the pure joy
of it all, so such tests—as well as such drugs—would be unnecessary, right?)

But utopia is not the hand we've been dealt. Sports today
are big business, even in the amateur ranks where money isn't
supposed to be an issue. It's the megamillions of dollars spent
by corporate America that keep the Olympics as big an event
as possible, with the huge profits generated by network cov-
erage, endorsements for Wheaties, Nike, and any other product gold-medal winners can endorse, and so on. When you
realize that Ben Johnson lost an estimated $30 million in
endorsements after his gold medal was revoked in Seoul in
1988, you start to get the picture.

So with all that money to be made, with all the fame and
glory to tap into, we know just how much is riding on success.
It doesn't take much thought to understand why athletes will
do anything they can to win. And they do!

"You May Win Once"

Whether we condone the use of steroids or not, it is clearly a
fact of life. Charlie Francis, who was banned from coaching
after Ben Johnson's positive drug test in 1993, recalls his decision to put several of his runners on controlled steroid regimens prior to the 1988 Olympics:

> Steroids could not replace talent, or training, or a
> well-planned competitive program. They could not
> transform a plodder into a champion. But they had
> become an essential supplement at the world-class
> level, an indispensable ingredient within a complex
> recipe. As I saw it, a coach had two options: He
> could face reality and plan an appropriate response,
> or he could bury his head in the sand while his ath-
> letes fell behind.[1]

Many coaches and trainers agree with Francis's assessment. Michel Karsten, a Dutch physician who prescribed steroids for athletes for over twenty-five years, says that he believes there may be some athletes who can win gold medals without taking drugs, but they are few in number. "If you are especially gifted," he says, "you may win once, but from my expe-

Ben Johnson lost an estimated $30 million in endorsements after being stripped of his medal and being banned from the sport in 1988. His coach, Charlie Francis (pictured), was banned from coaching and has written a book about the Olympic scandal.

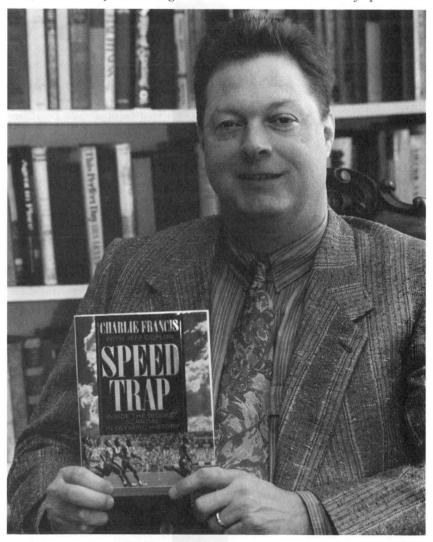

rience, you can't continue to win without drugs. The field is just too filled with drug users."[2]

Simply a Training Tool

To those who feel drug use soils the integrity of sports, it seems a dismal picture. One expert calls the use of steroids and other drugs "[t]he most serious threat to the Olympic ideal today. . . . The Olympics have in some ways become a mere proving ground for scientists, chemists, and unethical physicians."[3]

But to athletes who want to win, it's reality. For the athletes in many events—particularly track and field—steroids are simply a training tool, like free weights or vitamins. So what's the reaction among such athletes when various governing bodies in sports punish an athlete who uses these tools?

Anger, for one. Every athlete knows that for every one of his or her peers that is caught through drug testing, scores of others escape because their coaches have correctly calculated the number of days it takes for the drugs to be completely out of their systems. Or perhaps they escape because they are using certain "untraceable" drugs, of which there are many.

So the athletes who are caught are being told that they must obey rules that other athletes are breaking. Not only that, but the other athletes are the ones setting all the new performance records—the fastest time, the longest jump, the best throw. And these records —the drug-enhanced records—are the ones that the nonusers are told that they must surpass to become champions.

"You Can Never Set a World Record"

Nations like Canada that have decided to take a hard line on drugs are essentially taking their athletes out of world competition. As Francis insists, by strictly enforcing the steroid rules, Canada is telling their athletes, "You cannot make money in your chosen profession. You can never set a world record. You are barred from the big leagues."[4]

Even those who support the ban on steroids admit that the records set today in track and field events are most likely drug-enhanced. If ever all drugs *could* be banned, says one antisteroid physician, "at that point we should begin recognizing a completely new set of world and national records."[5]

But that will probably never happen. The users now seem always to be three jumps ahead of the testers, as it will undoubtedly remain in the future. What *will* happen is that the elite athletes will almost always be the ones who use steroids and other performance-enhancing drugs. True, athletes will not be *forced* to use steroids. The choice for each athlete will not be "Do I take drugs or not?" but "Do I want to compete on a national or international level or not?" Then the athlete trains accordingly.

For to compete without steroids today, especially on an Olympic level, is to be defeated before you even begin. As one physician attests,

> [Olympic athletes] would come to me and say, "Unless you stop the drug abuse in sports, I *have* to do drugs. I'm not going to spend the next two years in training—away from my family, missing my college education—to be an Olympian and then be cheated out of a medal by some guy . . . who is on drugs."[6]

The choice for competitive athletes, then, is really no choice at all.

1. Charlie Francis, *Speed Trap*. New York: St. Martin's Press, 1990.

2. Quoted in Michael Bamberger and Don Yaeger, "Over the Edge," *Sports Illustrated*, April 14, 1997.

3. Robert Voy, *Drugs, Sport, and Politics*. Champaign, IL: Leisure Press, 1991.

4. Francis, *Speed Trap*.

5. Voy, *Drugs, Sport, and Politics*.

6. Quoted in Bamberger and Yaeger, "Over the Edge."

CHAPTER 3

Should Drug Use in Sports Be Banned?

"We owe it to ourselves to demand that athletes are not cheaters, substance abusers, or criminals."

Performance-Enhancing Drugs Should Be Banned

"I don't think we can accept all the glory and the money that comes with being a famous athlete," said basketball star Karl Malone not long ago, "and not accept the responsibility of being a role model, of knowing that kids and even some adults are watching us and looking for us to set an example."[1]

I'm sure that there were people who rolled their eyes at Malone's words, just as I'm sure that there are many who feel that sports stars have no right to be examples of anything—except maybe how to do jump shots or slam dunks. After all, we live in a world where a twenty-one-year-old kid can demand—and get—a salary of $15 million a year to play basketball, or where a so-called amateur athlete can earn tens of thousands of dollars just for being seen in sweatshirts and shoes with a certain logo.

I'll admit that it's very easy to become jaded. We might even convince ourselves that some of those old ideas about athletes being heroes and role models are outdated, belonging to an era when things were much more simple. In such times, it never would have occurred to athletic governing bodies that athletes—professional or amateur—were using substances to help them gain an unfair edge over their opponents, substances that were harmful and, in some instances, could be fatal. It never would have occurred to people a generation or two ago that sports could be tainted in that way.

Is There a Place for Heroes?

Many today scoff at those old-fashioned ideas and say that even if the sports world was ever pure, it certainly isn't today. Editorialist Ellis Cashmore notes that those who still believe that sports are on a higher plane than the rest of life just haven't been paying attention—sports are just a flashy branch of big business. "Championships are prefixed with brand names," Cashmore says, "kits [uniform jerseys] are plastered with logos, performers shamelessly endorse products. . . . The marketplace brings with it imperatives, the central one of which is to win, not simply compete."[2]

Inarguably, commercialism has left its mark on sports. However, there is still an undeniable place within the world of sports for heroes, for fair play and honor. More than people in any other profession, athletes are viewed by many—especially young people—as role models.

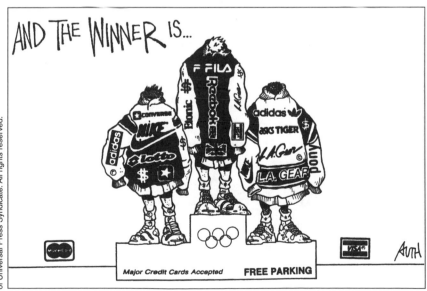

"Like it or not," writes one observer, "they have a power of influence on worshipful young fans multiplied by the huge factor of television—perhaps even more so among the minority poor, who have few other avatars of success to excite their hopes."[3]

For that reason alone, I think we owe it to ourselves to demand that athletes are not cheaters, substance abusers, or criminals.

"He Blew Carl Lewis' Doors Off"

Some argue that it's not really cheating when athletes use drugs, for it allows them to run, throw, jump, lift, or shoot better than those who don't use drugs. Take the example of Ben Johnson, the sprinter who was found to have used steroids in the 1988 Olympics and was subsequently banned from track.

Johnson's performance in Seoul was amazing—his run in the one hundred meters set a world's record. Young people who watched the event on television were wowed, and with good reason. And experts agreed that, as the news of Johnson's steroid use was announced, the drug got a lot of publicity—most of it very positive. As one professor of sports medicine recalls, "After Johnson got caught, a number of my colleagues agreed steroid use would increase. He was big, he was buff, and he blew [American rival] Carl Lewis' doors off. That's still the fastest time ever recorded."[4]

This is hardly the message we want to send to America's youth—that using steroids can turn an athlete into a superstar. But unless we as a society give wholehearted support for increasing bans on performance-enhancing drugs like steroids, that *is* the message young people will receive.

"I'm Sick of Watching Athletes Cheat"

It's time to call it what it is: cheating. A race won by a runner injecting illegal chemicals into his body to make him run faster just cannot be as important as one in which the participants play by the rules. As one Olympic expert writes,

> As a sports enthusiast . . . a world's record means
> nothing to me when I know chemical substances
> played a significant role in that achievement. I'm
> sick of watching athletes cheat their way onto the
> winner's podium at the Olympic Games. Moreover,
> I'm tired of seeing clean athletes, who sacrifice so
> much to earn a shot at the gold, fall short because
> they aren't using drugs to enhance their perfor-
> mances.[5]

Steroids and other similar drugs represent a major threat to the integrity of sports today. It is only by preserving this integrity that we can teach young people the value of competition, the importance of working and training and sacrificing to achieve a goal.

As former U.S. drug czar William Bennett says simply, "Athletes should be held to higher standards than other citizens."[6] By allowing athletes the choice of taking shortcuts, of using drugs instead of hard work to achieve muscle and speed, we are tacitly agreeing with the idea that the only value of sports is winning, and that the standards should be lowered. And if that should happen, we would all become the losers.

1. Karl Malone, "One Role Model to Another," *Sports Illustrated*, June 14, 1993.

2. Ellis Cashmore, "Run of the Pill," *New Statesman and Society*, November 11, 1994.

3. David Gelman, "I'm Not a Role Model," *Newsweek*, June 28, 1993.

4. Quoted in Skip Rozin, "Steroids: A Spreading Peril," *Business Week*, June 19, 1995.

5. Robert Voy, *Drugs, Sport, and Politics*. Champaign, IL: Leisure Press, 1991.

6. Quoted in Don Nardo, *Drugs and Sports*. San Diego: Lucent Books, 1990.

"Since when are we in the business of banning the use of things by competent people?"

Health Risks Should Not Be Used as an Excuse to Ban Steroids

One of the most frequently cited reasons for banning the use of steroids and other performance-enhancing drugs is that they pose a health risk. As former chief medical officer for the U.S. Olympic Committee Robert Voy remarks, "Because I am a physician and realize the dangers inherent in drug use, allowing athletes to use performance-substances is, in my mind, an irresponsible and completely unacceptable approach to creating a level playing field."[1]

Simply Paternalism

Let's forget, for the moment, that it is a fact that no significant dangers of steroid use have been proven. For the sake of argument, let's concede that an athlete may face some health risks by using performance-enhancing drugs. My comment, then, to Dr. Voy? "Baloney!"

I do not for a moment doubt Voy's sincerity in not wishing ill health on anyone; I only disagree with his feeling that it is up to him (or the Olympic Committee, or the National Football League, or whomever) to do something about it. Voy believes that performance-enhancing drugs pose a health risk to the users, but it does not naturally follow that they should be banned. Since when are we in the business of banning the use of things by competent people just because those things have the possibility of being a health risk?

To me it all smacks of paternalism, the notion that it is up to us as a society to protect people from themselves. It's an arrogant way of thinking, as though we somehow have a bird's-eye view of right and wrong, even when it comes to issues that are clouded.

The Health Police?

And to establish ourselves in the steroid issue as though we were a newly inducted regiment of the health police is absurd. If I were an athlete who used steroids in the course of my training, I would have some serious questions for people who wanted to ban them merely because they could pose a health risk.

For one thing, it seems as though society's concerns were applied very spottily. After all, plenty of behaviors that people choose to do could be considered health risks, but they are not banned. Aren't fatty foods such a health risk? Sports superstar Michael Jordan makes millions doing commercials in which he pushes Big Macs—a heart attack on a bun, as some physicians dryly refer to them. Where is the concern there? And what about smoking, or drinking? Athletes engage in these behaviors all the time, but we don't consider banning *them*.

One writer points out the curious contradiction this way:

> A female runner using oral contraceptives to regulate her period and so maximize her training and performance, or a chess player who smokes to calm his nerves are allowed to compete, despite taking [these substances] with known harmful consequences. But there is woe for anyone who takes cough [syrup] without carefully checking the label.[2]

It certainly seems as though society would demand a ban on all harmful substances, or potentially harmful substances, if it were truly committed to protecting the athletes.

Football, Boxing, and "the Yurchenko"

But that brings up a whole new area of dangers for athletes—the sports themselves! Some of the things athletes do are

Some sports are inherently dangerous to athletes. Gymnasts often must arch their backs to such an extent that the vertebrae are permanently ground down and damaged. Olga Korbut, pictured here in 1973, was struck with arthritis at age 27.

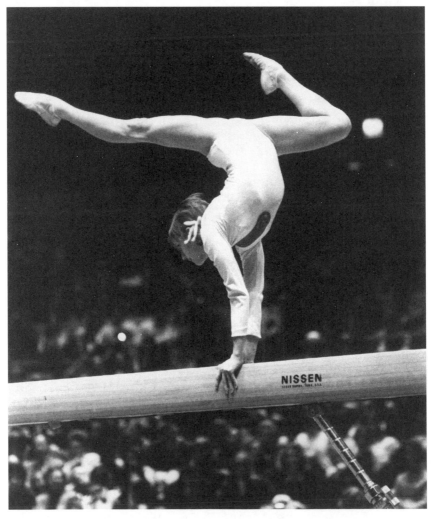

downright dangerous—or hasn't anyone else noticed? And if they're all noticing, where is the concern?

Are we concerned about the deaths from head injuries in diving or in football? Are we concerned at the beatings men give one another in the boxing ring—a popular spectator sport? It was said of Muhammad Ali, one of the greatest boxers of all time: "The man who took punches for twenty-seven years, twenty-one as a pro, is punch-drunk and brain damaged."[3]

Or how about women's gymnastics? Perhaps the most graceful and aesthetically pleasing sport to the spectator, but the training and competition are grueling on young bodies. Look at Olga Korbut, who once charmed Olympic audiences with her grace and style. By the time she was twenty-seven, Korbut had become riddled with arthritic pain brought on by her gymnastics.

As one coach critically notes,

> We permit adolescent girls to attempt dangerous maneuvers like "the Yurchenko," a backward launch onto the vaulting horse (which landed one American in a coma at the Tokyo World Sports Fair in 1988), or to arch their backs to the point where they grind down—and permanently deform—soft, young vertebrae.[4]

Arrogance and Hypocrisy

Clearly, we are not worried enough to change sports to eliminate the risks. Medical ethics professor Norman Fost points to the example of a foul known as "roughing the passer," which occurs when a quarterback is hit after the whistle or hit with more aggression than necessary.

It's a particularly worrisome foul, simply because the quarterback is more vulnerable to injury than some of the more heavily padded contact players. The possibilities for serious injury are rife, says Fost, but perpetrators receive only mild penalties. "If the consequence . . . were a three point penalty," observes Fost, "the practice would disappear, and far more disability would be prevented than has been attributed to steroids by even their most severe critics."[5]

No, let us not show our arrogance, our hypocrisy, by pretending we are protecting our athletes as we make rules prohibiting them from using steroids. Our health police's unwillingness to protect these young men and women in other, far more damaging, activities is proof enough of that.

1. Robert Voy, *Drugs, Sport, and Politics*. Champaign, IL: Leisure Press, 1991.

2. Ellis Cashmore, "Run of the Pill," *New Statesman and Society*, November 11, 1994.

3. Howard Cosell, quoted in Hank Nuwer, *Sports Scandals*. New York: Franklin Watts, 1994.

4. Charlie Francis, *Speed Trap*. New York: St. Martin's Press, 1990.

5. Norman C. Fost, "Ethical and Social Issues in Antidoping Strategies in Sport," in *Sport . . . The Third Millennium/Sport . . . Le Troisieme Millenaire*, ed. Fernand Landry, Marc Landry, and Magdeleine Yerles. Quebec: Presses de L'Universite Laval, 1991.

"If all athletes have access to steroids, where is the unfair advantage?"

Unfair Advantage Should Not Be Used as an Excuse to Ban Steroids

In the 1972 Olympic Games an American pole vaulter named Bob Seagren tried to get the Olympic Committee to agree to allow him to use a fiberglass pole. His pole was certainly an improvement on the ones other vaulters used at the time; fiberglass was lighter and stronger, and Seagren found it gave him far more maneuverability in his jumps.

The committee agreed with Seagren that the fiberglass pole seemed to be superior to traditional poles. For that very reason, however, they prohibited Seagren from using it to compete in the Olympic Games that year. None of the other vaulters had had access to the fiberglass pole, and thus the advantages it provided meant an unfair advantage to Seagren. The ban was lifted four years later in Montreal, when it was determined that access to the fiberglass pole had been equalized.

No Fairness in Sports

The idea of what is these days commonly called a "level playing field" is a noble one, and should not be questioned. That

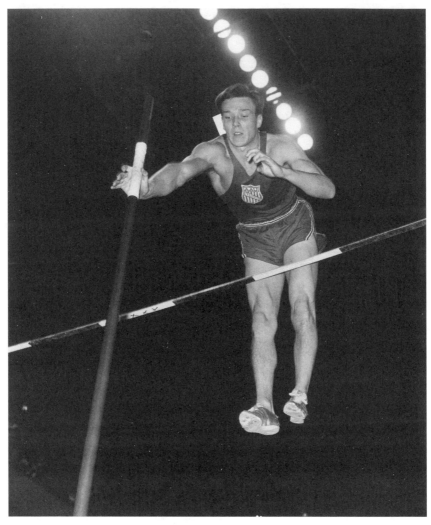

Robert Seagren was not allowed to use a fiberglass vaulting pole in the 1972 Olympics because the judges thought it would give him an unfair advantage over the rest of the pole vaulters who used wooden poles. This rule was repealed four years later.

competition should be on equal terms for all is not questioned by any thoughtful person. For one runner to have a lane that is dry and smooth, while one has mud and potholes is unfair. For one gymnast to have access to resin before using the parallel bars, while others must do their routines with sweaty palms is unfair. These are the conditions of competition, and they must be consistent for each participant.

But the idea of fairness in training—what each competitor brings to the competition in his or her physical makeup, skills, and abilities (*including* the use of steroids and other performance-enhancing drugs)—that idea of fairness is ludicrous. For example, as one writer observes,

> Were you a runner, born in Bradford, following home Yobes Onidieki in a 5,000 metres race, you may wonder what difference it would have made if you, like your opponent, had been born and raised in Kenya, where the altitude encourages a naturally high hemoglobin count—a boon for middle-distance runners.[1]

And what about the obvious advantages of a short build for a high diver or keen eyesight for an archer? Are those things unfair? Any clear-thinking individual would respond "no," for these are merely differences in athletes' genetic endowments. The line becomes a little fuzzier, however, when the question of what is fair moves from endowments to training choices.

"Whatever They Can to Win"

There is an infinite range of choices athletes can make in their training regimens. Hundreds of thousands of dollars are spent in the pursuit of just the right diet, just the right strength training. "Performers can boost their performances," one writer argues, "by recruiting top coaches, nutritionists, acupuncturists; they can use state-of-the-art equipment and, if they can afford it, train in optimal climes."[2]

Far from being unfair, this is the nature of sport—to gain an edge, however slight, over one's opponents. And make no mistake, in events that are measured by fractions of seconds, a tiny edge can make all the difference. As one Olympic coach notes, "As long as hundredths of seconds translate into millions of dollars and blinding celebrity, athletes will do whatever they can to win."[3]

Often what they do—at least in the United States—is take advantage of a large budget and high-tech equipment. The 1990 American volleyball team, for instance, found that they could improve the leaping ability of the players by consulting with kinesiologists and biomechanists, as well as using million-dollar computers to measure each athlete's movement styles.

Where Is the Line?

But at what point do we say an athlete's choice crosses the line from "innovative training" into the "cheating" territory? Why is the admitted steroid use of a runner like Canada's Ben Johnson cheating, when these other, high-tech efforts, many not available to poorer nations, are not? If all athletes all have access to steroids, where is the unfair advantage? Where is the line being crossed? If an athlete chooses *not* to use performance-enhancing drugs in his or her training, that is a choice—in the same way that a particular kind of diet is a choice, or the kind of strength-training machine used for workouts.

"From Nautilus Machines to Gatorade"

Princeton bioethics professor Norman C. Fost has found nothing in his research that would indicate that using steroids is much different from using certain legal substances that boost athletic performance. He finds it puzzling that steroid use has attracted so much negative attention.

> The widespread use of anabolic steroids by athletes is upsetting to many people, but it is not clear why. The objection that steroids provide an "unnatural" assist to performance is inchoate. Many of the means and ends which athletes use and seek are unnatural. From Nautilus machines to . . . Gatorade, their lives are filled with drugs and devices whose aim is to maximize performance.[4]

As steroids continue to be outlawed, and athletes who exhibit traces of the substances are censured and humiliated, officials are inviting well-deserved protests, especially if they continue to give the reason as "unfair advantage."

1. Ellis Cashmore, "Run of the Pill," *New Statesman and Society*, November 11, 1994.
2. Cashmore, "Run of the Pill."
3. Charlie Francis, *Speed Trap*. New York: St. Martin's Press, 1990.
4. Quoted in Michael Bamberger and Don Yaeger, "Over the Edge," *Sports Illustrated*, April 14, 1997.

CHAPTER 4

Should Athletes Be Tested for Drugs?

"Drug testing is a big waste of time. It's an exercise in futility."

Drug Testing Athletes Is Futile

I'm only the messenger, so please be civil. I am in no way condoning the use of drugs in the Olympic Games or any other athletic contest, amateur or professional. But it has got to be said: Drug testing is a big waste of time. It's an exercise in futility.

At the 1996 Summer Olympic Games held in Atlanta, the machinery of the drug-testing procedure was hailed as state-of-the-art by experts. As one reporter wrote, just days before the opening of the games,

> The IOC's [International Olympic Committee's] doping team will deploy handpicked technicians and three $700,000 high-resolution mass spectrometers, said to be five to 10 times more sensitive to the telltale traces of banned drugs than any other device available. The process is pricey—perhaps $800 per test.[1]

"Comically Ineffective"

A superficial look at the results of the drug testing in Atlanta might have convinced some that drug use was down among Olympic athletes. After all, the high-tech equipment produced only two sanctioned positive tests—down from five at the 1992 Olympics and twelve in the Los Angeles 1984 Olympics.

75

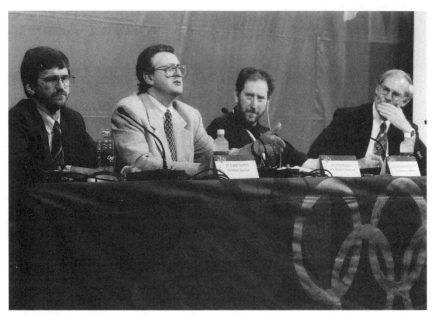

During a press conference, doctors answer questions about the drug-testing program used during the 1996 Olympics.

Untrue, most Olympic insiders would reply. Coaches, athletes, administrators, and even steroid traffickers say that the Atlanta Olympics, like other Olympics of the last fifty years, "was a carnival of sub-rosa experiments in the use of performance enhancing drugs . . . [and] the drug-testing effort was . . . comically ineffective."[2]

The low number of positives, they say, had far more to do with the ability of athletes and trainers to outwit the machines than with a sudden dip in drug usage. "The testers know," said one Olympic medical official, "that the [drug] gurus are smarter than they are. They know how to get in under the wire."[3] The director of a prestigious drug-testing lab agrees wholeheartedly. "The sophisticated athlete who wants to take drugs," he explains, "has switched to things we can't test for."[4]

No Test for EPO

New drugs are certainly a big part of the problem. EPO, a bioengineered form of a hormone called erythropoietin, is one such drug. It belongs to the class of drugs known as performance enhancers; EPO increases red-blood-cell counts and allows athletes to absorb more oxygen, thereby boosting their endurance. Investigators have found that at least twenty deaths in recent months can be linked to the use of EPO, and they have warned athletes to avoid it.

A chemist transfers a urine sample to prepare it for drug testing. This is the same procedure that is used during the Olympic games.

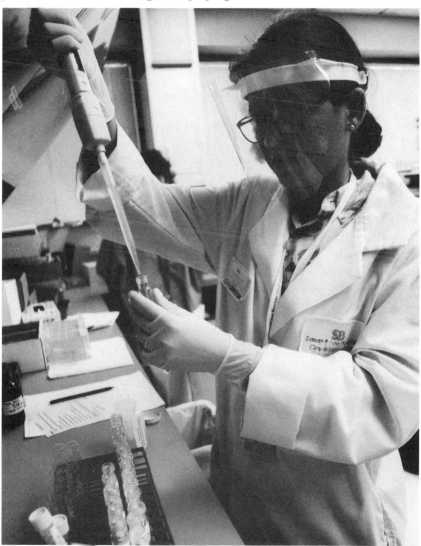

For all the dangers associated with it, however, the drug *can* work. The unfortunate part for athletic governing committees is that, unlike for steroids, there is no test that can detect EPO's presence in blood or urine. Since the drug started becoming common with runners and other athletes for whom endurance is a valued commodity, athletic officials have been noticing an amazing increase in overall performances. One Canadian distance runner says that he has been amazed at the rate of improvement in the past five years. "The red flag goes up when someone suddenly takes 11 seconds off a world record, which is pretty unheard-of by most runners. You kind of think, 'Holy Cow, how the hell are these guys doing this?'"[5]

Designer Drugs and Drug Gurus

Many athletes have their own "drug gurus"—part chemists, part trainers. After the gurus purchase illegal performance enhancers for their clients, they chemically alter them just enough so that they are not traceable. As researchers Michael Bamberger and Don Yaeger explain:

> Each type of steroid has a unique signature that shows up in the urine of a user. Because drug testers look only for the signatures of commercially available steroids, a steroid whose signature has been changed will be much more difficult to detect. For an athlete using that altered steroid, passing a drug test becomes a breeze.[6]

Unfortunately for the integrity of athletics, this claim is no exaggeration. Gurus themselves admit that they haven't seen a mass spectrometer yet they haven't been able to fool. "No athlete I've ever helped has tested positive," brags one, "and I've helped hundreds."[7]

Tricks of the Trade

Athletes and trainers alike know that it is a wise precaution to discontinue the use of steroids a few weeks before a competition. (Even with designer drugs, which supposedly cannot be traced, many athletes prefer to stop use a week or two before an event, just to be safe.) Once an athlete stops using steroids, they are gradually flushed out of the system until no trace of them remains.

Athletes and trainers also know that the benefits of such drugs diminish slightly when they are discontinued, so the trick is to find that little window of opportunity—close enough to use so that the benefits of speed, muscle, and endurance remain, but not too close to the event that they might be discovered in a drug test. Testing officials report that some athletes would prefer not to discontinue the steroids before an event, and instead resort to more devious methods to avoid detection.

Women occasionally show up for testing with condoms containing "clean" urine concealed in the vagina. Some athletes drink vinegar beforehand, which can interfere with a test's accuracy. And some athletes have been known to urinate before an event, "insert a catheter up his or her urethra, and then use the equivalent of a turkey baster to squeeze someone else's urine into his or her bladder."[8] It's gruesome—but sports today are big business and big money, so risks like these are worth it for the serious athlete.

The Stuff of Which Nightmares Are Made

And suppose the occasional athlete *does* test positive—what then? Drug testers know all too well that a positive can have all sorts of questions attached to it. Could the sample have been contaminated by faulty refrigeration? Was the sample tampered with by someone from a rival team? Was it an error in the procedure, or a glitch in the machine?

And what happens then? Sometimes follow-up tests have a different result, sometimes not. An athlete could be suspended, but this happens rarely. Some athletic organizations are afraid of lawsuits, which have become extremely plentiful.

Add to this the basic fact that many athletic organizations—including the Olympics—do not want to see offenders get caught, for high-profile athletes are what draws spectators, sponsors, and television time.

Clearly, drug testing athletes is an expensive, inexact procedure, which cannot guarantee accurate results. And even those results are questionable. It's unfortunate, but true—drug testing athletes as it exists today is an exercise in futility.

1. Rae Corelli, "The Drug Detectives," *MacLean's*, July 22, 1996.

2. Michael Bamberger and Don Yaeger, "Over the Edge," *Sports Illustrated*, April 14, 1997.

3. Quoted in Bamberger and Yaeger, "Over the Edge."

4. Quoted in Bamberger and Yaeger, "Over the Edge."

5. James Deacon, "A Phantom Killer," *MacLean's*, November 27, 1995.

6. Bamberger and Yaeger, "Over the Edge."

7. Quoted in Bamberger and Yaeger, "Over the Edge."

8. Bamberger and Yaeger, "Over the Edge."

"If we are going to take the high road where drugs and sports are concerned, we've got to be serious about our testing for those drugs."

Drug Tests Can Work

Much has been said recently about the rampant drug use in amateur and professional sports. The discussions seem to be accompanied by a great deal of hand wringing and head shaking, a sure sign that no solution is forthcoming. In fact, what has been proposed as a sort of "nonsolution" is that we do nothing at all. Instead of enforcing the ban on certain drugs and saying that to use them is unfair, harmful, and promotes the wrong kind of competition in sports, it has been suggested more than once that we allow the drugs because it is too difficult to test athletes for them.

"A Race Among Pharmacologists"

I agree that the testing we now do is imperfect, but to lift the ban we have placed on certain drugs seems awfully defeatist. It's a little like deciding we will no longer have speed limits on our highways because speeding is so common and police officers are so few. Why not just give in and let people decide how fast they want to go?

No, if we stop trying to enforce rules in athletics, we get chaos. If we stop testing for drugs, we are sending a message that their use is acceptable. Then, says the head of one IOC-accredited drug-testing lab, "we would just have a race among pharmacologists to find better and stronger drugs. Now at least they [the athletes] have to worry about being detected."[1]

Unfortunately, it doesn't seem these days that they worry much at all. Many athletes and coaches privately (and sometimes publicly) have talked about the rampant use of performance-enhancing drugs in their sports.

Negative Outlooks

Some insiders scoff at the idea that drug testing works, and to be truthful, it does seem sometimes that the odds are certainly stacked against honesty. Former British Olympian David Jenkins, who himself was jailed for black-market distribution of illegal drugs, scoffs at the idea that sports—especially international events such as the Olympic Games—could be cleaned up. "Sport is no longer," he claims. "What is this illusion of innocence, of fair play, of good fun for all? That exists as a dream in people's minds."[2]

The problem, of course, is that far too much is at stake these days for sport to be pure. Individual athletes see the enormous amounts of money to be made—even at the amateur level. "In 1964, an Olympic gold medal might have been a nice piece of memorabilia," sighs one Olympic coach. "Today that medal can be worth millions."[3]

Governments themselves are a problem, too. Many of them use athletic contests such as the Olympics to prove the superiority of their politics over other nations. (We saw plenty of that among the Communist Eastern bloc countries in past decades.) Two researchers worry about "biologically prepared and pharmacologically manipulated individuals performing to bolster the prestige of participating governments or ideologies."[4] It's little wonder that many athletes would do anything—risk anything—just to win.

Who Does the Testing?

"We need an outside organization, not the track federations, to test for drugs," maintains U.S. track superstar Carl Lewis.

"They felt that they had too much at risk and couldn't afford to have top athletes getting caught on drugs. That would make the whole sport look bad."[5]

Former U.S. Olympic Committee officer Robert Voy agrees:

> When an international hero such as Ben Johnson is exposed for cheating, everyone—I mean *everyone*—feels repercussions from this blow. The sport federations lose money. They lose public interest and support. They are forced to face sharp, intense scrutiny from the media. Thus, many officials seem more willing to turn their backs on the problems, sweep them under the rug, and avoid an exposé rather than become a laughingstock before the world.[6]

For precisely this reason, the choice of *who* does the drug testing is critical. Why on earth are we entrusting the job to the national sports groups, when losing a key athlete because of a positive drug test would be devastating? Do we really think that these groups will be fastidious when testing their own superstars? Talk about the fox guarding the henhouse!

It makes far more sense to have a testing agency that answers to no government, to no team. And, since the testing is such an expensive undertaking, have *all* participating nations chip in to pay for it. And what if a country refuses to pay its share? It doesn't compete—period.

When Should We Test?

Once we've decided on the *who* of testing, we should take a long look at *when* it needs to be done. Just as most insiders agree on the need for impartial, nongovernment testing for drugs, they also agree that it is too easy for drug users to avoid being caught when they are tested the day of the event.

Steroids and other performance-enhancing drugs are *training* drugs. They are of benefit to athletes the weeks and months before competition; the effects are still evident long after the athlete stops a cycle of usage. As one expert says,

"Any athlete with a brain and a calendar can use anabolic-androgenic steroids to benefit today with little or no fear of detection."[7]

So the trick is to test the athletes during training, when drug use would be more likely—if it were an issue at all. Although several plans have been suggested, Dr. Voy's seems the most realistic. He suggests that sports administrators should begin requiring a twelve-week registration deadline before *all* major competitions. Explains Voy, "Those athletes registered to compete should be informed and then subjected to short-notice (48- to 72-hour) drug tests at any time within that twelve-week period, beginning with a test at registration."[8]

Even though many drugs can disappear from the system within three or four weeks, athletes would have to carefully weigh the benefits of use. Since a user would have to discontinue fifteen or sixteen weeks before a competition, most advantages of the drugs would surely be minimal.

Everything to Gain

I agree wholeheartedly with Douglas McKeag, a former investigator for the National Collegiate Athletic Association drug surveys, who says that these drugs "may constitute the single most significant threat to the integrity of sports in this country, and drug use and abuse certainly constitutes the most significant threat to the future of sport."[9]

If we are going to take the high road where drugs and sports are concerned, we've got to be serious about our testing for those drugs. At this point, it seems that there is very little to lose—and everything to gain.

1. Quoted in Michael Bamberger and Don Yaeger, "Over the Edge," *Sports Illustrated*, April 14, 1997.

2. Quoted in Tom Donohoe and Neil Johnson, *Foul Play: Drug Abuse in Sports*. Oxford: Basil Blackwell, 1986.

3. Charlie Francis, *Speed Trap*. New York: St. Martin's Press, 1990.

4. Donohoe and Johnson, *Foul Play*.

5. Carl Lewis, *Inside Track: My Professional Life in Amateur Track and Field*. New York: Simon and Schuster, 1990.

6. Robert Voy, *Drugs, Sport, and Politics*. Champaign, IL: Leisure Press, 1991.

7. Voy, *Drugs, Sport, and Politics*.

8. Voy, *Drugs, Sport, and Politics*.

9. Quoted in James E. Wright and Virginia S. Cowart, *Anabolic Steroids: Altered States*. Carmel, IN: Benchmark Press, 1990.

Appendix A

Views of Drugs and Sports

Document 1: A Host of Unexpected Symptoms

In his book Drugs, Sport, and Politics, *former chief medical officer for the U.S. Olympic Committee Robert Voy includes a list of the known side effects experienced by athletes and others who take anabolic steroids.*

- Acne: serious cystic types that leave permanent scars on the face, body, and trunk
- Nervous tension, aggressiveness, and psychotic states; paranoia; and antisocial behavior
- Increased sex drive after initial use, but decreased sex drive after repeated use (often leading to psychologically caused impotence)
- Breast development in males, also known as gynocomastia (a permanent effect)
- Gastrointestinal and leg muscle cramping
- Headaches, dizziness, and high blood pressure
- Burning and pain while urinating
- Bizarre testicular or scrotal pain
- Premature male baldness (particularly alarming among 17-year-olds)
- Excessive body and facial hair growth among women
- Atrophy of testicles and decreased sperm production
- Prostate enlargement, causing urination to be difficult
- Enlargement of the clitoris, the female organ analogous to the male penis (usually irreversible and may require surgical removal)
- Deepening of the voice (permanent in women)
- Stunted growth among adolescents, basically due to premature stoppage of the expected growth of long bones

Document 2: A Patriotic Drug

One of the people most distressed about the prevalence of steroid abuse among athletes was Dr. John Ziegler, the man known as the father of anabolic steroids. In Bob Goldman and Ronald Klatz's book, Death in the Locker Room: Drugs and Sports, *they describe Ziegler's introduction of the drugs to U.S. athletes as being done out of a spirit of patriotism.*

The introduction of anabolic steroids to U.S. athletes, by Dr. Ziegler's own account, was done out of patriotism following a dark period in U.S. history. In 1956, the decade of "McCarthyism," with its fears of Soviet expansion in Europe, was just ending. On the international sporting scene, the cold war was anything but cold. The Olympics had become the arena where winning was believed by many to be a reflection of the correctness of the winner's political system. Dr. Ziegler, like many others, was a victim of this misplaced athletic chauvinism. His intention was not to do harm, but to help his country out of loyalty. Doc Ziegler, a former World War II hero, was highly decorated, and had special training in general surgery, neurology, geriatrics, and physical and nuclear medicine, [and] was outraged by the success of the Soviets, who he discovered were using male hormones to build weight and power, while our boys were slogging along with diets and workouts alone.

While in Vienna, Dr. Ziegler had drinks with a Soviet team physician who admitted that they were using hormones. Said Dr. Ziegler, "I felt the Russians were going to use sports as the biggest international publicity trick going—and strength sports especially. They saw it as a political advantage 100 percent." Dr. Ziegler went to the Ciba Pharmaceutical Company . . . and together they worked out a program to develop an anabolic steroid to give to weight lifters, the first to try it out, at the York (Pennsylvania) Barbell Club.

The problem was that the weight lifters loved the drugs and weren't satisfied to stay on the recommended dosages. Said Dr. Ziegler, "They figured if one pill was good, three or four would be better, and they were eating them like candy." The news of anabolic steroids spread . . . and soon drugs and stories of drugs became the chief topic of conversation at training camps and the subject of articles in all of the sports magazines.

So sadly, Dr. Ziegler's work, that he had viewed as American, can-do science at its best, providing Americans with the tools to win, became distorted, misunderstood, and abused. Dr. Ziegler learned early, and seeing the dangers signaled by anabolic steroids run wild, he ceased his advocacy of them, but it was too late [to stop them from being used]. The magic growth genie wouldn't go back in the bottle.

Document 3: Psychotic Behaviors and Steroid Use

Scientists have identified certain behavioral changes among steroid users, ranging from uncontrolled aggression to deep depression. In his book Macho Medicine: A History of the Anabolic Steroid Epidemic, *William N. Taylor includes the following statements from a mother and father whose son died as a result of these behavioral changes.*

On August 7, 1989, we found our beautiful 18-year-old son hanging from a tree by our front door. . . . We found five bottles of Dianabol [a commonly used steroid] in his car after his death. . . . He began using them (anabolic steroids) the summer before his senior year in high school to prepare himself for football. . . . He gained thirty pounds in a short time and his muscles began to appear very defined. . . . We were unaware of the psychological effects of steroid use. We now know that Eric's symptoms and subsequent depression and suicide were a result of withdrawal from the drugs [anabolic steroids]. . . . Eric had exhibited many episodes of abnormal aggressiveness during the year before his death. Once, when someone cut him off, Eric flew into a rage, pulled the man over, and beat him up. A week before his death, he pulled two men over near a shopping center and beat one of them. Several times Eric became enraged at his family members over inconsequential events. . . . There was no way to predict what would set him off. Once, he pounded dents into the hood of the family car. He alternated between rational and irrational thoughts. . . . Eric was an amazing kid. He never took any other drugs, nor did he drink more than an occasional beer at a party. . . . We suspected steroid use and advised him to stop. . . . These drugs are deadly, and we want that fact known.

Document 4: Seeking Scapegoats?

In his paper "Ethical and Social Issues in Antidoping Strategies in Sport," Norman Fost argues that sports have evolved into something very different from what they were in the past, and that society is overreacting in its condemnation of athletes who have used performance-enhancing drugs. This paper is contained in Sport . . . The Third Millennium, *edited by Fernand Landry, Marc Landry, and Magdeleine Yerles.*

Something is surely amiss in sports. If amateurism means competing for the "love of the thing," it seems to have faded as the sole basis of athletics and of Olympic competition long before the present time. Exploitation, politics, and economic considerations increasingly dominate sports throughout the world, as the third millennium draws near. In the face of these complex and seemingly intractable problems, it is perhaps understandable that scapegoats would be sought as a distraction. The extent and intensity of the vilification cast on Ben Johnson would lead one to believe he has violated some moral principle that is at the bedrock of society.

I fail to see what, if any, purely moral principle he violated. He *broke* a rule and most assuredly risked losing (and indeed lost) his medal as a consequence. But the rule is not based on any coherent moral principle the demonstration of which has been offered by those who had promulgated the rules. And whatever moral principles might be involved, such as gaining unfair advantage, or preventing harm, are most everywhere violated in far more obvious and worrisome ways, with little comment or apparent effort at correction.

Document 5: A Lucrative Steroid Business

Although steroids have been on the U.S. federal controlled-substance list since 1991, they are evidently still as available as ever before. Their legal manufacture has been restricted in the United States, but as Skip Rozin explains in this excerpt from his article "Steroids: A Spreading Peril," in Business Week, *other countries are picking up the slack.*

While legal drug sales have doubled in the past five years, to $71 billion, legitimate steroid sales in the U.S. are down to about $3 million annually at wholesale. That's less than half the figure for 1989, before they were controlled, says Susan Koch of IMS America, a pharmaceutical marketing research firm.

Foreign opportunists have rushed to satisfy illegal demand in the U.S. Steroids' new popularity has spurred production in Greece, India, Poland, and Spain according to the Drug Enforcement Administration (DEA), and recent investigations indicate activity in South Korea. But the results of a six-month *Business Week* inquiry point to Europe and Mexico as primary sources for the international steroid traffic, a trade generating as much as $750 million a year.

Dr. Tomas Buril, former director of the Czech Republic's national drug intelligence service, observes that political upheaval in Eastern Europe has allowed clandestine steroid labs to flourish. With privatization of the pharmaceutical industry, Buril says, many of the rigid controls of the communist regimes have disappeared, and drug traders have capitalized on cracks in the system.

Russia's Drug Control Dept. reports that steroids reach the black market right from factories and warehouses, to be sold openly on the street. And Buril says that steroids stockpiled by the former Red Army, which encouraged their use, have just disappeared. Of grave concern are potentially more hazardous animal growth hormones coming out of Bulgaria. "It is quite easy to convert these products for human consumption," says Ladislav Koukal, an Interpol officer in the Czech Republic.

Document 6: The Psychology of Steroid Use

In their book Warning: Drugs in Sports, *Andrew Ferko, Edward Barbieri, and G. John DiGregorio discuss what they feel are the incorrect views of sports that help athletes rationalize the use of performance-enhancing drugs.*

Today, a very disconcerting area of inappropriate drug use is drug taking by athletes to enhance their performance in competition.... All of this drug-taking activity by athletes is called *doping in sports*. It is being done in the name of excellence to perform in competition. The ultimate goal of the drug-taking athlete is to win at any cost and those costs may be greater than the athlete realizes.... Anything short of winning to some is losing, and when this occurs, feelings that they have failed themselves, their teammates, their coaches, and their parents arise.

The emotions of failure, ineptness, lack of ability, depression, and desperation overcome them. Any avenue available to increase their athletic ability now becomes acceptable. The chant of "no one likes a loser" rings loud and clear in their minds. Reasonable judgments become clouded and rationalization comes to the forefront. Anything that it takes to win is "right" to them. Academics are pushed aside; relaxation becomes a waste of time. Relationships suffer and excessive training becomes a total obsession.

Thoughts of drug usage that can increase performance and stamina, or that can reduce fatigue and pain, now become appropriate in their minds; these thoughts are then turned into actual drug-seeking behavior. This last part of the athlete's conscious decision is relatively easy because drugs are readily available to them through a variety of means. They will use any lie or distortion of symptoms, if necessary, to obtain their "golden crutches" and the chance to excel.

However, the bottom line is that athletes who have become obsessed with winning and employ drugs to achieve their goal were actually losers and cheaters from the very beginning . . . they just never realized it. . . . Sports allows individuals to demonstrate their natural athletic talents, and to help their team in competitive events. To play sports is supposed to be fun and enjoyable. It is not an arena to obtain individual selfish goals.

Document 7: Encouraged by a Coach

In 1989, hearings were conducted before the Senate Committee on the Judiciary concerning the link of drugs and sports in the United States. One of those who testified was former national track champion Diane Williams, who detailed her use of steroids and their effects on her. The following excerpt from that testimony is from Macho Medicine: A History of the Anabolic Steroid Epidemic *by William N. Taylor.*

I was able to train longer and harder, which ultimately improved my performance. Immediately I developed acne and light pigmentation on my face. I was a woman who suddenly became strong like a man. . . . I had no menstrual period . . . and certain masculine features appeared, like a mustache and fuzz on my chin. My clitoris, which is a penis equivalent, started to grow to embarrassing proportions. My vocal cords lengthened to a deeper voice. And a muscular pattern of hair growth appeared. Steroids affected my sexual behavior. . . . In women, the production of testosterone is quite low and the androgen is synthesized by the adrenal gland and is indirectly responsible for the women's sex drive.

My following athletic achievements were a result of the steroid Dianabol. I am currently a collegiate record holder of the women's 100 meters with a time of 10.94. I was second at the Athletic Congress National Championships in Indianapolis, June 1983. I was a bronze medalist at the first world championship in Helsinki, Finland during the summer. I received my first major commercial endorsement with Life magazine. . . . [The coach] supplied me with more Dianabol and furthermore, he charged me a fee of 10 cents to 25 cents a pill, depending on whatever he felt was appropriate. And at the time I had a little bit more money that I made, sponsorship money from winning the bronze medal.

There are approximately 45 to 50 women on a team (who used steroids) . . . 40 percent of the 1988 [Olympic] team had tried it at least.

And one of the psychological effects that I had at the time is I really believed that I could not run fast after [I stopped taking] steroids. I did not believe that I had the natural ability to run fast. . . . I have really, really, been brainwashed by this coach.

Document 8: Student-Athlete Consent Form

Each year, college athletes must sign a form declaring their understanding of the National Collegiate Athletic Association (NCAA) drug-testing program and their willingness to participate. The following is part of the form in which athletes agree that they will be tested for drugs.

By signing this part of the form, you certify that you agree to be tested for drugs.

You agree to allow the NCAA, during this academic year, before, during or after you participate in any NCAA championship or in any postseason football game certified by the NCAA, to test you for the banned drugs listed in Executive Regulation 1-7(b).

You reviewed the procedures for NCAA drug testing that are described in the NCAA Drug Testing Program brochure.

You understand that if you test positive (consistent with NCAA drug-testing protocol) you will be ineligible to participate in postseason competition for at least 90 days.

If you test positive and lose eligibility, and then test positive again after your eligibility is restored, you will lose postseason eligibility in all sports for the current and next academic year.

You understand that this consent and the results of your drug test, if any, will only be disclosed in accordance with the Buckley Amendment consent.

| _____ | _____ |
| date | Signature of student athlete |

| _____ | _____ |
| date | Signature of parent if student athlete is a minor |

Document 9: The Olympic Ideal

Those who favor banning steroids and other drugs from sports often cite the integrity and morality of sport as an important virtue. In the following excerpt from his article "Ethical Issues of Drug Use in Sport" (contained in Athletes at Risk: Drugs and Sport, *edited by Ray Tricker and David L. Cook), Ralph A. Vernacchia discusses the framework for sports ethics, the ideals of the ancient Olympic Games.*

According to the Olympic ideal, the pursuit of athletic excellence is to be balanced, complemented, and realized by placing equal emphasis upon the intellectual, spiritual, social, and ethical growth and development of the aspiring athlete.

Ultimately, the athlete must evaluate how he or she achieved success and recognition, for there is a distinct difference between a winner and a champion. Champions are remembered and valued not solely for what they achieved but how they earned their recognition, and in some cases, how they responded in defeat. Although there are many winners in athletics, there are truly only a few champions. The champion is humble and compassionate in victory, dignified in defeat, and resolved to be the best in future competitive situations.

The achievement orientation of sport administrators, coaches, and athletes should reflect their desire to be winners and champions, while at the same time realizing that although one cannot always win, they can always attain the satisfying self-actualizing benefits of a championship effort. It is, therefore, the educational charge and challenge of both coaches and athletes to achieve *victory with honor*.

Document 10: Dishonor Among Athletes

One of the arguments for enforcing drug bans on athletes is that athletes are role models for our society In her article "Sports Have No Standards Left," for Conservative Chronicle, *Mona Charen laments the fact that we do not expect more from athletes—and in fact that we tolerate their dishonorable acts.*

George Steinbrenner, owner of the Yankees, has just offered more than $800,000 to Darryl Strawberry—drug addict, wife beater and tax evader. The man deserves a second chance, Steinbrenner explains.

Of course, Strawberry has already had many, many second chances—chances offered without any real evidence of repentance. Pete Rose was thrown out of baseball forever and forbidden entry into the Hall of Fame (perhaps justly) for gambling, Strawberry has assaulted two wives, cheated on his taxes and taken illegal drugs repeatedly, and yet is offered more second chances than a cat has lives.

Of course, Steinbrenner is not anybody's idea of a moral exemplar. He would probably offer a contract to Saddam Hussein if he could bat .350. . . .

We haven't lost our sense of shame entirely in this country. But we've certainly begun applying it in peculiar ways. When Marge Schott [then owner of the Cincinnati Reds baseball team] uttered ethnic insults, she was (deservedly) written out of polite company, but when Michael Jackson included ethnic insults about Jews on his latest album, he was treated with kid gloves. Darryl Strawberry can cheat on his taxes, take drugs, and beat his wives—and still count on understanding and indulgence from employers and the public.

Well, sports figures are not role models, say worldly sports columnists. They're just athletes.

But if your dentist did what Strawberry did, would you take your children to him? How about your pharmacist? Or your grocer? In point of fact, the role model question is a red herring. It isn't a question of leading children astray, but simply enforcing some sense of shame and honor on everyone.

We have come to a lamentable pass when shame is not feared and when dishonor is seen only as an opportunity for synthetic "redemption."

Document 11: Official Testing Procedure

In their article "Drug Testing: History, Philosophy, and Rationale," in Athletes at Risk: Drugs and Sport, *edited by Ray Tricker and David Cook, James Merdink and Bruce Woolley explain the safeguards built into the system of drug testing. This excerpt explains the protocol of the collection of the urine sample used to test an athlete.*

The collection procedure used by the NCAA and the U.S. Olympic Committee was designed with strict chain-of-custody to ensure sample integrity throughout the collection and testing procedures. The sample identity is known only to the governing bodies.

The athlete is usually notified of the test immediately after competing, and is given one hour to report to the collection facility. An athlete signature form is filled out with a personal history and a declaration of all drugs taken recently (prescription or over-the-counter). This declaration is used to identify possible banned compounds before the actual testing of the sample. A collection container is randomly selected to prevent any deliberate tampering. Collection of the urine specimen takes place under the direct observation of a trained attendant. The athlete must produce a urine specimen of at least 100 mls [milliliters]. Sodas and water are available for those who cannot produce the required volume of urine.

The athlete chooses two sample containers which will become known as the A- and B-samples. The A-sample is tested immediately, while the B-sample is frozen for later analysis in the event of a legal challenge. The urine is poured from the collection container into the two sample containers, while retaining a small amount of a pH and specific gravity test. These two tests ensure that an unadulterated specimen has been collected. Unacceptable specimens are rejected and another specimen will be collected. The samples are capped and a numerical code attached to each container. It is important that the athlete verify that all numbers on the sample containers and the paperwork match. The samples are sealed into shipping containers and sent to the laboratory for testing.

Document 12: Random Testing Won't Work

Many experts agree that one of the weaknesses of drug testing today is its predictable timing; athletes can stop taking a drug weeks before an event and traces of the drug will disappear so there is no detection. Some have called for random testing, although Dr. Robert Voy explains why that might not work in this excerpt from his book Drugs, Sport, and Politics.

Some countries already have this type of program. The Scandinavians—the Swedes and the Norwegians in particular—do such unannounced testing. Believe me, it works, at least when they are able to surprise the athlete. That is very difficult to do, though, because the testing officials seldom are able to make all of the planned athlete contacts.

I really can't envision a program like that working in the United States. First of all, a program like this would never withstand the pressure of organizations like the American Civil Liberties Union and various players unions—with good reason. This SWAT-team approach to drug testing would be a gross violation of individual rights. I just can't justify dragging athletes out of their beds in the middle of the night to ask them to urinate in a bottle. This is not only degrading but also a violation of the U.S. Constitution.

Imagine also, if you will, the enormous expense of trying to track down an athlete who might be in Rome one week, Tokyo the next, and New York the next week, all in an attempt to run one urinalysis test. You can understand why such a system wouldn't work; doping control agencies would exhaust their entire budgets going after only several dozen athletes.

Also, the communications network of athletes is extraordinary. For example, I once tested Swedish athletes at American universities. Sometimes, the minute the drug crew hit the campus front gates, athletes were already in the next county. It proved to be a tremendous financial burden trying to pin down athletes targeted for testing.

APPENDIX B

Facts About Drugs and Sports

- Although cocaine is considered the most addictive recreational drug, it has become common among athletes as both a recreational and a performance-enhancing drug.

- Bodybuilders estimate that between 98 and 100 percent of athletes in their sport use steroids.

- One of the newcomers on the drug market, known as hGH (human growth hormone), carries risks, too. Some users develop jutting foreheads, prominent cheekbones, and an elongated jaw.

- Erythropoietin, or EPO, can increase endurance by as much as 25 percent. As of 1997 it is not detectable in urine drug tests.

- After China's women's swim team won twelve of sixteen gold medals at an international meet in 1994, seven of the women tested positive for drugs.

- Drug tests for steroids allow a man to have a testosterone/epitestosterone (a natural hormone found in urine) ratio of 6:1, even though most men have a ratio of 1.3:1 or lower. Thus, experts say, it is possible for a male athlete to artificially increase his ratio to 6:1 and still avoid detection.

- Women are allowed the same 6:1 ratio, even though experts say it is unheard-of for a woman to have a testosterone level of more than 2.5.

- The use of steroids is reputed to have spread to every sport, from baseball and soccer to basketball and football.

- Eighty percent of male track and field Olympic athletes have used steroids at one time. Thirty percent of college basketball players have used them. And in 1990 it was estimated that 75 percent of NFL athletes used steroids on a regular basis.

- One of the concerns today is the use of so-called brake drugs, which stunt the growth and maturation of athletes. Eastern European coaches and trainers have been accused of giving brake drugs to their female gymnasts to keep their girlish bodies from developing.

- Michelle Smith, the Irish swimmer who won three gold medals at the 1996 Olympics, has been informally accused of using steroids. Smith did pass drug tests, and both she and her coach deny drug use; however, many members of the media and other swim teams believe otherwise.

- Half the teenagers who use steroids start before they are sixteen.

- The typical teen steroid user is male and white; however, teenage girls between fifteen and eighteen represent the fastest-growing user group.

- Government officials estimate that there are more than ten thousand outlets for illegal performance-enhancing drugs in the United States.

- The price of steroids on the black market ranges from $15 to $120 per bottle.

- The top-selling steroid on the black market is Clenbuterol, intended for veterinary use.

- There is even a high degree of drug use among athletes who participate in events such as shooting, archery, billiards, and snooker. The drugs of choice are "beta-blockers," which slow the heartbeat and steady the hand.

- One performance enhancer that is difficult to test for is called "blood packing" or "blood doping." This involves the removal of a few hundred milliliters of blood, which is stored for several weeks. Before the competition, the blood is transfused back to the athlete. Because of the added red blood cells and oxygen in the blood, the athlete has better endurance and more energy.

STUDY QUESTIONS

Chapter 1

1. What is meant by the term *stacking*? Why does the author of Viewpoint 1 consider it dangerous?

2. In what ways does a steroid user risk developing a Dr. Jekyll and Mr. Hyde personality? What research has been done confirming the existence of 'roid rage?

3. Does the author of Viewpoint 3 agree with Coach Vince Lombardi's assessment of winning? Do you? Why or why not?

4. Why does the author of Viewpoint 4 feel the death of Lyle Alzado is not proof that steroids are dangerous? Do you think longtime steroid users such as Sergio Oliveira can aid the debate about the health risks of steroids? Why or why not?

Chapter 2

1. Do you think coaches who urge steroids and other performance-enhancing drugs on their athletes believe there are health risks?

2. In what ways do the authors of Viewpoints 1 and 2 differ in their assessment of athletes' responsibilities? Do you agree more with one or the other? Explain your answer.

3. Do you agree with the author of Viewpoint 3 who says that drugs are just another training tool? Why or why not?

Chapter 3

1. Do you agree with former U.S. drug czar William Bennett that athletes should be held to higher standards than other citizens? How might Charlie Francis, Ben Johnson's former coach, respond to Bennett?

2. What does the author of Viewpoint 2 mean by "paternalism" as it applies to athletics and drug use?

3. What is meant by the idea of a level playing field? Do steroids or other drugs change a level playing field into one that is uneven? Why or why not?

Chapter 4

1. The author of Viewpoint 1 feels that drug testing is so inefficient that it should be stopped. Do you agree?

2. Do you agree with David Jenkins about the state of sports today? Would Carl Lewis agree or disagree with Jenkins's statement?

ORGANIZATIONS TO CONTACT

American College of Sports Medicine
PO Box 1440
Indianapolis, IN 46206
(317) 637-9200

This organization is a good source of information on the risks of performance-enhancing drugs such as steroids and human growth hormone.

International Amateur Athletic Federation (IAFF)
17 Rue Princesse Florestine
BP 359
MC 98007 Monco Cedex, Monaco
377-9310-8888

The IAFF is the international governing body of athletics, with 180 member federations around the world. It produces its own list of doping control regulations and distributes an antidrug booklet for young athletes.

National Collegiate Athletic Association (NCAA)
6201 College Blvd.
Overland Park, KS 66211-2422
(913) 339-1906

The NCAA is the national administrative body overseeing all inter-collegiate athletics. It publishes up-to-date information on regulations (including those concerning drugs) for college athletes in the United States.

National High School Athletic Coaches Association (NHSACA)
PO Box 5020
Winter Park, FL 32793
(407) 679-1414

The NHSACA seeks to promote cooperation among coaches, school administrators, the press, and the public. It holds seminars in sports medicine and promotes educational programs on drug abuse awareness.

U.S. Olympic Committee (USOC)
1750 East Boulder St.
Colorado Springs, CO 80909
(719) 632-5551
Like other national Olympic committees around the world, the USOC publishes codes of ethics to which Olympic athletes are expected to adhere. The USOC also has compiled a detailed list of drugs athletes are banned from using in competition.

FOR FURTHER READING

Gayle Olinekova, *Winning Without Steroids*. New Canaan, CT: Keats Publishing, 1988. Highly readable; helpful bibliography.

Angela Patmore, *Sportsmen Under Stress*. London: Stanley Paul, 1986. Good information on the ways athletes rationalize drug use.

Katherine Talmadge, *Drugs and Sports*. Frederick, MA: Twenty-First Century Books, 1991. Easy reading; good section on psychoactive drug use among athletes.

Ray Tricker and David L. Cook, eds., *Athletes at Risk: Drugs and Sport*. Dubuque, IA: Wm. C. Brown, 1990. Good combination of very specific details about various drugs and interesting text.

Dave Tuttle, *Forever Natural: How to Excel in Sports Drug-Free*. Venice, CA: Iron Books, 1990. Interesting chapter on man-made hormones.

Melvin H. Williams, *Beyond Training: How Athletes Enhance Performance Legally and Illegally*. Champaign, IL: Leisure Press, 1989. Helpful explanations of uses and side effects of various drugs used by athletes.

Works Consulted

Books

Edward F. Dolan, *Drugs in Sports*. New York: Franklin Watts, 1986. Easy text, with helpful information on brake drugs.

Tom Donohoe and Neil Johnson, *Foul Play: Drug Abuse in Sports*. Oxford: Basil Blackwell, 1986. Informative section on the future of drug testing, especially in international events.

Andrew P. Ferko, Edward Barbieri, and G. John DiGregorio, *Warning: Drugs in Sports*. West Chester, PA: Medical Surveillance, 1995. Helpful information on amphetamines.

Norman C. Fost, "Ethical and Social Issues in Antidoping Strategies in Sport." In *Sport . . . the Third Millennium/Sport . . . Le Troisieme Millenaire*, ed. Fernand Landry, Marc Landry, and Magdeleine Yerles. Quebec: Presses de L'Universite Laval, 1991, pp. 479–85. Contains numerous articles on a wide variety of subjects related to sports and society.

Charlie Francis, *Speed Trap*. New York: St. Martin's Press, 1990. Readable account of Ben Johnson's experience with drugs.

Bob Goldman and Ronald Klatz, *Death in the Locker Room: Drugs and Sports*. Chicago: Elite Sports Medicine Publications, 1992. Good section on human growth hormones; excellent glossary.

Carl Lewis, *Inside Track: My Professional Life in Amateur Track and Field*. New York: Simon and Schuster, 1990. Fascinating "inside" information on drugs and the world of track and field.

Don Nardo, *Drugs and Sports*. San Diego: Lucent Books, 1990. Easy reading; helpful overview on those who profit from drug use among athletes.

Hank Nuwer, *Sports Scandals*. New York: Franklin Watts, 1994. Readable; good index and bibliography.

———, *Steroids*. New York: Franklin Watts, 1990. Good information on how athletes obtain steroids; helpful index.

Lisa Angowski Rogak, *Steroids: Dangerous Game*. Minneapolis: Lerner Publications, 1992. Very easy reading; helpful glossary and resource list.

Mark Sabljak and Martin H. Greenberg, *Sports Babylon: Sex, Drugs, and Other Dirty Dealings in the World of Sports*. New York: Bell Publishing, 1988. Good chapters on Len Bias and Dwight Gooden.

William N. Taylor, *Macho Medicine: A History of the Anabolic Steroid Epidemic*. Jefferson, NC: McFarland, 1991. Helpful information on the limits of drug testing.

Robert Voy, *Drugs, Sport, and Politics*. Champaign, IL: Leisure Press, 1991. Good section on the history of drug use in sports.

Gary I. Wadler and Brian Hainline, *Drugs and the Athlete*. Philadelphia: F.A. Davis, 1989. Excellent appendixes.

James E. Wright and Virginia S. Cowart, *Anabolic Steroids: Altered States*. Carmel, IN: Benchmark Press, 1990. Excellent section on current methods of drug testing.

Periodicals

Jose Antonio, "What the Media Missed on 'Roid Rage," *Muscle & Fitness*, January 1997, p. 48.

"At Issue: Should Schools Have the Right to Randomly Test Athletes for Drug Use?" *CQ Researcher*, September 22, 1995, p. 841.

Michael Bamberger, "Under Suspicion," *Sports Illustrated*, April 14, 1997, p. 72.

Michael Bamberger and Don Yaeger, "Over the Edge," *Sports Illustrated*, April 14, 1997, p. 60.

Ellis Cashmore, "Run of the Pill," *New Statesman and Society*, November 11, 1994, p. 22.

Stephen Chapman, "Living Under the Unblinking Eye of Big Brother," *Conservative Chronicle*, July 12, 1995, p. 4.

Mona Charen, "Sports Have No Standards Left," *Conservative Chronicle*, July 12, 1995.

Rae Corelli, "The Drug Detectives," *MacLean's*, July 22, 1996, p. 28.

James Deacon, "A Phantom Killer," *MacLean's*, November 27, 1995, p. 58.

Bill Dobbins, "Steroids: Are They Heaven . . . or Are They Hell?" *Muscle and Fitness*, October 1996, p. 106.

"The First and Only Time I Used Steroids," winning contest entry, Belle International, November 1997, p. 1.

David Gelman, "I'm Not a Role Model," *Newsweek*, June 28, 1993, p. 56.

Jeff Hollobaugh, "Track Is Losing the War on Drugs," *ESPN Sports-Zone*.

"IOC Removes Seven Drug-Testing Labs from Its Approved List," *NCAA News*, April 12, 1989, p. 5.

James J. Kilpatrick, "The Athlete and the Drug Test," *Conservative Chronicle*, June 22, 1994, p. 15.

Karl Malone, "One Role Model to Another," *Sports Illustrated*, June 14, 1993, p. 84.

Steve Marantz, "Addiction by Distraction," *Sporting News*, May 27, 1996, p. 10.

Barry Maron, "Sudden Death in Young Athletes: Lessons from the Hank Gathers Affair," *New England Journal of Medicine*, July 1, 1993, p. 55.

Jack McCallum, "Fair or Foul?" *Sports Illustrated*, March 20, 1995, p. 26.

Leigh Montville, "Flora and Furor," *Sports Illustrated*, September 19, 1994, p. 40.

Mary Nemeth, "Scandal: Act 2," *MacLean's*, March 15, 1993, p. 18.

Joseph Nocera, "Bitter Medicine," *Sports Illustrated*, November 6, 1995, p. 74.

Sergio Oliveira, "The Steroid Problem: 'Roid Truth from a Man Who Knows," *Musclemag*, September 1995, p. 165.

S.L. Price, "Up in the Air," *Sports Illustrated*, March 27, 1995, p. 48.

Skip Rozin, "Steroids: A Spreading Peril," *Business Week*, June 19, 1995, p. 138.

———, "Steroids and Sports: What Price Glory?" *Business Week*, October 17, 1994, p. 176.

Joannie M. Schrof, "Pumped Up," *U.S. News & World Report*, June 1, 1992, p. 54.

Rick Silverman, "I Was a Teenage Science Project," *Muscle & Fitness*, April 1997, p. 200.

Tony Snow, "Olympics Have Become a Megabucks Spectacle," *Conservative Chronicle*, July 31, 1996, p. 31.

Tom Verducci, "The High Price of Hard Living," *Sports Illustrated*, February 27, 1995, p. 16.

George F. Will, "Students Get Lawyers, Authorities Get No Respect," *Conservative Chronicle*, July 2, 1995, p. 7.

INDEX

ABOUT THE AUTHOR

Gail B. Stewart is the author of more than eighty books for children and young adults. She lives in Minneapolis, Minnesota, with her husband, Carl, and their sons, Ted, Elliot, and Flynn. When she is not writing, she spends her time reading, walking, and watching her sons play soccer.